Dr Richard Petty
where he obtained
degree in Physiol
behavioural Research Centre in Boston, USA, in 1976 where he became interested in patients with emotional and language disorders. As a Research Fellow in Neurology at the Princess Margaret Clinic he was personally involved with migraine and headache sufferers, which led him to treat his patients at the Charing Cross Hospital with medical acupuncture. He has also spent several years investigating different forms of complementary medicine, and is currently a member of the Research Council for Complementary Medicine.

Dr Richard Petty has taught both undergraduate and postgraduate level medicine and has published many articles on various medical subjects. He is currently Senior Registrar in General Medicine at the Northwick Park Hospital and the Clinical Research Centre in Harrow.

Dr Tom Sensky qualified as a biochemist and obtained a Ph.D at London University. He then studied medicine, qualifying from University College Hospital, London. He pursued psychiatric training at the Maudsley Hospital in London and has since become a member of the Royal College of Psychiatrists.

Dr Sensky is now lecturer and honorary Senior Registrar at Charing Cross Hospital in London. He has collaborated with Dr Petty on several research projects and they have between them published over eighty medical and scientific papers.

Also by Dr Richard Petty
Migraine and Headaches

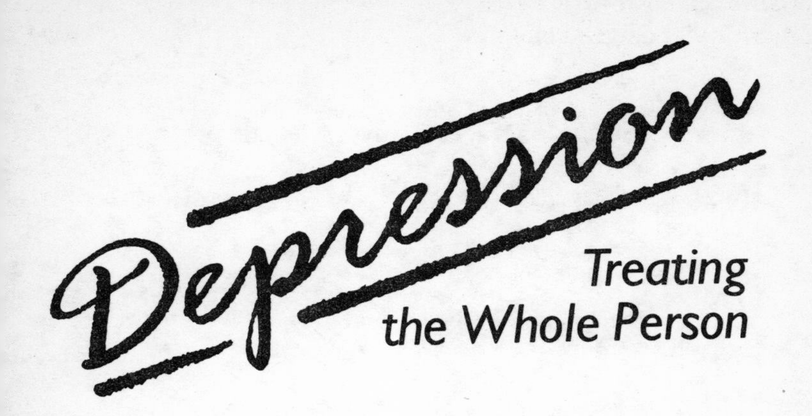

Dr Richard Petty and
Dr Tom Sensky

London
UNWIN PAPERBACKS
Boston Sydney Wellington

First published by Unwin Paperbacks 1987
This book is copyright under the Berne Convention. No reproduction without permission. All rights reserved.

UNWIN® PAPERBACKS
40 Museum Street, London WC1A 1LU, UK

Unwin Paperbacks
Park Lane, Hemel Hempstead, Herts HP2 4TE, UK

Allen & Unwin Australia Pty Ltd,
8 Napier Street, North Sydney, NSW 2060, Australia

Unwin Paperbacks with the Port Nicholson Press
PO Box 11-838 Wellington, New Zealand

© Dr Richard Petty and Dr Tom Sensky 1987

British Library Cataloguing in Publication Data

Petty, Richard
Depression: healing the whole person.
1. Depression, Mental—Treatment
I. Title II. Sensky, Tom
616.85'2706 RC537
ISBN 0-04-616031-0

Made and printed in Great Britain by
The Guernsey Press Co. Ltd., Guernsey, Channel Islands.

Contents

Introduction

Almost everyone would say that they knew what it was like to be depressed. For most of us, depression is no more than a vague feeling of sadness, but for others it becomes a specific state needing help and treatment. In these people, depression can often produce a whole host of physical and mental symptoms, from constipation to thoughts of suicide. Indeed, of all the people who consult their doctor some 10 per cent can be recognised as depressed.

The last few years have seen a quiet revolution in people's awareness about health and disease. For perhaps the first time, the idea of taking some personal responsibility for restoring and maintaining health has become a major concern for an enormous number of individuals. It seems paradoxical that this movement has developed at a time when the powers of conventional medicine have become even greater. There is also another apparent paradox — the idea that in some way the desire to take responsibility for oneself when unwell cuts across the concept of society caring for those who are in need of care and support.

The depressed person usually has no wish to read books and one of the symptoms of depression is an inability or unwillingness to do anything constructive for oneself. It is at this time that family and friends can be of enormous help, but in order to provide assistance of any sort, they must have access to reliable, up-to-date information about the nature of depression and the various forms of treatment which are available. Also, we have often been told by people who have recovered from depression that they are keen to learn precisely what happened to them and, in particular, to do what they can to avoid the same thing happening in the future. This book is written to address such questions. It is not intended to be a totally comprehensive account of depression and should supplement the advice given by your doctor, rather than substitute for it.

Although we deal with the conventional approaches to diagnosis and treatment, we are going to discuss at some length a number of alternative or unconventional approaches to treating depression. This is not because we are as yet convinced that all these treatments help but because patients and their relatives often ask us about such treatments. It is an area about which, until now, the available information has been the most inaccurate. We shall consider a variety of different alternative therapies but we must make it clear that we do not endorse any particular one of these.

It is important to stress that we are in no way underestimating the value of conventional approaches to the treatment of depression, and we regard it as vital that any form of treatment a person opts for is undertaken with the knowledge and approval of his or her doctor. Many people contemplating alternative medicine for the first time are concerned that such a move will alienate their doctor and that they will have to give up the familiar territory of conventional medicine if they pursue alternative treatments.

Also it must be remembered that these different approaches to treatment are not mutually exclusive. It is perfectly reasonable, and in fact desirable, to continue with both conventional treatment and the alternative approach simultaneously. The last few years have also seen a major change in the attitudes of many members of the medical profession. Although many doctors remain sceptical about the value of the alternative therapies, they are nowadays far more likely to agree to a supervised trial of some different approach and no one should fear that a visit to an alternative practitioner means burning one's boats with conventional doctors. And, as we shall show, there is indeed some early evidence that some of the alternative therapies can be very helpful to some people.

Finally, a word about our use of the term 'alternative therapies'. There are well over a hundred different such therapies. Far from all representing one point of view, they represent a vast number of different philosophies and techniques. Many people now favour the term 'complementary therapies' to suggest that they should work together with conventional medicine. We have decided in this book to use the older term, simply because many of the therapies have not yet proved their value, but we very much hope to see a time when these therapies can become truly complementary. Many of our patients and some of our colleagues have made the first steps towards this, and it is to them that this book is respectfully dedicated.

DEPRESSION

CHAPTER ONE

What Is Depression?

Albert was 70 years old and had worked as a watchman for the same firm for twenty-three years. As he grew older, both he and his wife found his shiftwork increasingly stressful and demanding, but he took great pride in the fact that he had never needed to take time off work through illness. Like his parents, both of whom had died of 'old age', Albert had remained well all his life. Always an active man, he had been slightly wary of retirement, but with his wife's encouragement, he had planned to redecorate their home and to spend more time with their grandchildren. Two years after his retirement, his wife unfortunately suffered a massive stroke and died shortly afterwards. His children were surprised how well Albert seemed to adjust to his wife's death. However, three years later, just after the date of Albert's wedding anniversary, his family began to notice a gradual change in him. He declined his daughter's invitation to spend Christmas with her family and became increasingly withdrawn, reluctant even to talk on the telephone as he had previously enjoyed doing. He lost interest in his family and nothing seemed to give him pleasure. He began to spend his days moping about the house, doing less and less. He paid little attention to his appearance and sometimes didn't shave for days. He lost his appetite and couldn't be bothered to prepare meals. His clothes began to look increasingly baggy as he lost weight. He awoke each morning at about 3 o'clock and was then unable to fall asleep again, despite feeling exhausted all the time. He dreaded those early hours, which to him somehow seemed worse than any other time of day.

His family watched all this with increasing concern. What they found most difficult to understand was that he had developed an irrational concern that he would shortly be arrested by the police. Some fifteen years earlier, the warehouse at which he had worked was broken into while he was on duty, though he discovered the thieves in time to raise the alarm. Nothing was taken and he was commended for his swift action. Now, he insisted to everyone that the burglary had been successful and that the police had recently come to suspect that he had conspired with the burglars. Nothing could dissuade him from this view. His part in apprehending the thieves had been described at the time by the local newspaper, but even when confronted with his newspaper cuttings, he insisted that they were completely wrong, adding that this may have been a deliberate attempt to extract a confession out of him. He insisted that he was worthless and deserved to be 'put away'. He saw no future for himself. By the time Albert's family finally persuaded him to seek help, he had lost more than 2 stones in weight and was becoming increasingly reluctant to eat or drink. His doctor arranged his admission to hospital for treatment.

Faced with life's inevitable difficulties and hurdles, we all become miserable from time to time. For most of us, this low mood does not last long and causes little interference in our lives. We may recognise things we can do to cheer ourselves up, to try to distract ourselves from the causes of our misery. For example, we might launch ourselves into some other activity, like a new hobby, or go on a shopping spree, or socialise more than usual. When we meet friends who feel in a low mood, we offer them similar advice. When we feel miserable in this way, we may even describe ourselves as 'depressed'. In this context, 'depression' is merely the description of a particular *mood* state, synonymous with feeling sad or miserable.

Albert's depression was an altogether different experience. For one thing, his low mood was not only severe but also persistent. He felt utterly without hope. As many families do under such circumstances, Albert's children initially responded to him as though he were merely sad, urging him to 'pull himself together', to take more interest in himself and in the family. In fact, the more they tried to cheer him up, the more he withdrew into himself. Although Albert's misery was profound, his depression involved a great deal more than this; he suffered weight and appetite loss, disturbed sleep, and was distressed by thoughts which, although very real to him, appeared irrational to other people. There are other people like Albert who, when they become very depressed in their mood, show similar disturbances of emotion, thought, sleep, and so on. All these features together make up one form of *syndrome* of depression.

A syndrome is a collection of features (or symptoms) which together characterise an illness. Consider, for example, a child who begins to feel unwell, with headache and poor appetite and one to two days later develops a high temperature and begins to experience pain on chewing or swallowing, accompanied by swelling under his jaw. This particular time sequence and pattern of symptoms suggests that the child has mumps, which can be confirmed by looking for further features of this condition. Should depression be considered an illness like mumps? This issue is complex and certainly remains controversial. Some have argued that all 'mental illness' is artificially created by doctors or by society. Our view, shared by most doctors, is that it is sometimes, although not always, appropriate to view depression as an illness. We shall return to this theme again.

Albert's depression was severe and incapacitating, causing his family and himself much distress. Few people who have known someone as depressed as Albert would have difficulty seeing this condition as an illness, for which 'treatment' or 'help' should be sought. Fortunately, relatively few people become as incapacitated by depression as Albert.

What, then, are the features of the syndrome of depression from which Albert was suffering? As we shall see, his is only one of several types of depression. In this particular form of depression, certain changes in bodily function are characteristic. Usually, weight falls (accompanied by a diminished appetite) but some people tend to eat much more when they become depressed, putting on weight. Sleep is disturbed, with early morning wakening as the characteristic pattern, leaving one feeling exhausted rather than refreshed after sleep. In women, menstrual irregularities are common, and periods may even cease temporarily; this happens when there has been marked weight loss. Loss of libido (sex drive) is also common together with other disturbances of sexual function. There is also a tendency to feel at one's worst first thing in the morning; this time-dependent pattern which repeats itself daily is called diurnal variation. A person with depression may be very agitated or withdrawn and slowed down in thought and action like Albert. Conversation becomes very difficult, as the depressed person will sometimes take a long while to answer even the simplest question and may even become completely mute. He may move about so little that bed sores develop. Doctors refer to these particular bodily disturbances as 'biological' or 'vegetative' features of depression. It is worth stressing here that, although these symptoms occur in depression, each of them may have many causes. Thus although loss of sexual drive, for example, is a feature of depression, depression is only one of many causes of loss of libido.

Depression like Albert's also involves numerous psychological features. There is a specific alteration in mood. Sadness, which is common to most forms of depression, can be severe and persistent. Some people with depression find themselves crying much more than usual, often for no apparent reason. Others find themselves unable to cry, and complain that they are unable to feel any emotion. They recognise that they want to love their partners and families but find themselves incapable of doing so. Loss of energy is a common complaint. There is also loss of enjoyment, which may be so severe that there is nothing from which the depressed person is able to derive pleasure. Life assumes a totally hopeless quality and there appears to be no future. The individual feels worthless and may blame him or herself for long-forgotten mishaps in his life for which he was not directly responsible.

The illogical ideas Albert developed are also a feature of severe depressions of this type. These are ideas that are manifestly false and not shared by other people under similar circumstances. They are held with unshakeable conviction, even though the person concerned is able to understand and reason about other things quite normally. Such ideas are called delusions. To others, someone who has a delusion may appear to be very stubborn, but it is important that being deluded embraces much more than simple stubborness. Often, the illogical nature of delusions is strikingly obvious. However, there are times when it is difficult to tell with certainty whether a particular idea is false or not, for example, an extra-marital affair which may or may not have happened thirty years previously. Albert's idea about the burglary was clearly false; it not only remained with him but also clearly distressed him a great deal. Yet he was unresponsive to reassurance. This is characteristic of delusions and often very difficult for friends and family to understand. Our next case vignette illustrates this.

Michael had been brought up in a strict Roman Catholic household, though, in his 50s, he stopped attending church. Some years later, he became very depressed, refusing to eat or drink anything, and insisting that he had sinned by forsaking the church and that it was the will of God that he should die. Nothing that the local priest, as well as members of his family, said could dissuade him from this view. In fact, their attempts to reason with him only made everyone feel worse. Some weeks later, after his depression had been successfully treated, Michael rapidly gained a stone in weight and completely abandoned his former guilt, although he remained ambivalent in his attitude towards the church and his faith.

A particular danger for people who are as depressed as Albert or Michael is the risk of suicide. Investigations of the histories of people who have committed suicide reveal that probably some 70 per cent of them suffered from depression. These figures are tragic bearing in mind that depression is usually eminently treatable.

The pattern of depression so far described, with the biological or bodily features already noted, is known as *endogenous depression*; 'endogenous' means 'arising from within' — it used to be held that this type of depression arose in the absence of any obvious precipitants. However, this is no longer considered so; in Albert's case, for example, his depression seemed to follow the date of his wedding anniversary. The term 'endogenous' is still used to describe the collection of features listed above.

When delusions are present, the depression is sometimes then called *psychotic depression*. Someone who has delusions is, by definition, no longer fully in touch with reality because he is unable to understand that his beliefs are false. He cannot even concede that his beliefs *may* be false. This failure to recognise that one's beliefs (and sometimes also one's experiences) conflict with reality is the hallmark of psychotic conditions. As we have already noted, it may sometimes by very difficult to tell whether or not a person's beliefs are contrary to reality.

We have chosen to begin by describing this type of depression because its features, and often its severity, make it easier to recognise than other forms. Relatively few people, however, will ever experience this type of depression. By contrast, many will be able to identify with some of the features in the next case history.

Eileen was 25 years old, recently separated from her husband and struggling to bring up her two young children, Darren (aged 5) and Tracey (aged 2). Eileen had two younger sisters but no brothers, and her husband, Paul, was her parents' first son-in-law. Eileen's parents thought the world of him and had done all they could to encourage the marriage. Paul worked as a heavy-goods vehicle driver, a job that kept him away from home for days at a time, while Eileen had given up her job as a trainee supermarket manageress when she married. At first, the marriage had been very happy, but Eileen had never been enthusiastic about Paul's work; she missed him while he was away and found herself worrying that he might be involved in a road accident. When Paul was away, Eileen found the children difficult to cope with; Darren especially became very demanding and had also started wetting the bed. When Paul was home, Eileen and he would often argue about the children and about his job. She did her best to persuade him to find a job with regular hours nearer home, while he insisted that his present job paid well and that the family needed the money he brought in. Paul found it difficult to understand his wife's anxiety and their arguments became more frequent and increasingly heated. Eventually, after they had come to blows one evening, Paul decided to return to live with his parents to let things cool off. The rest of the family took his departure very badly; Darren

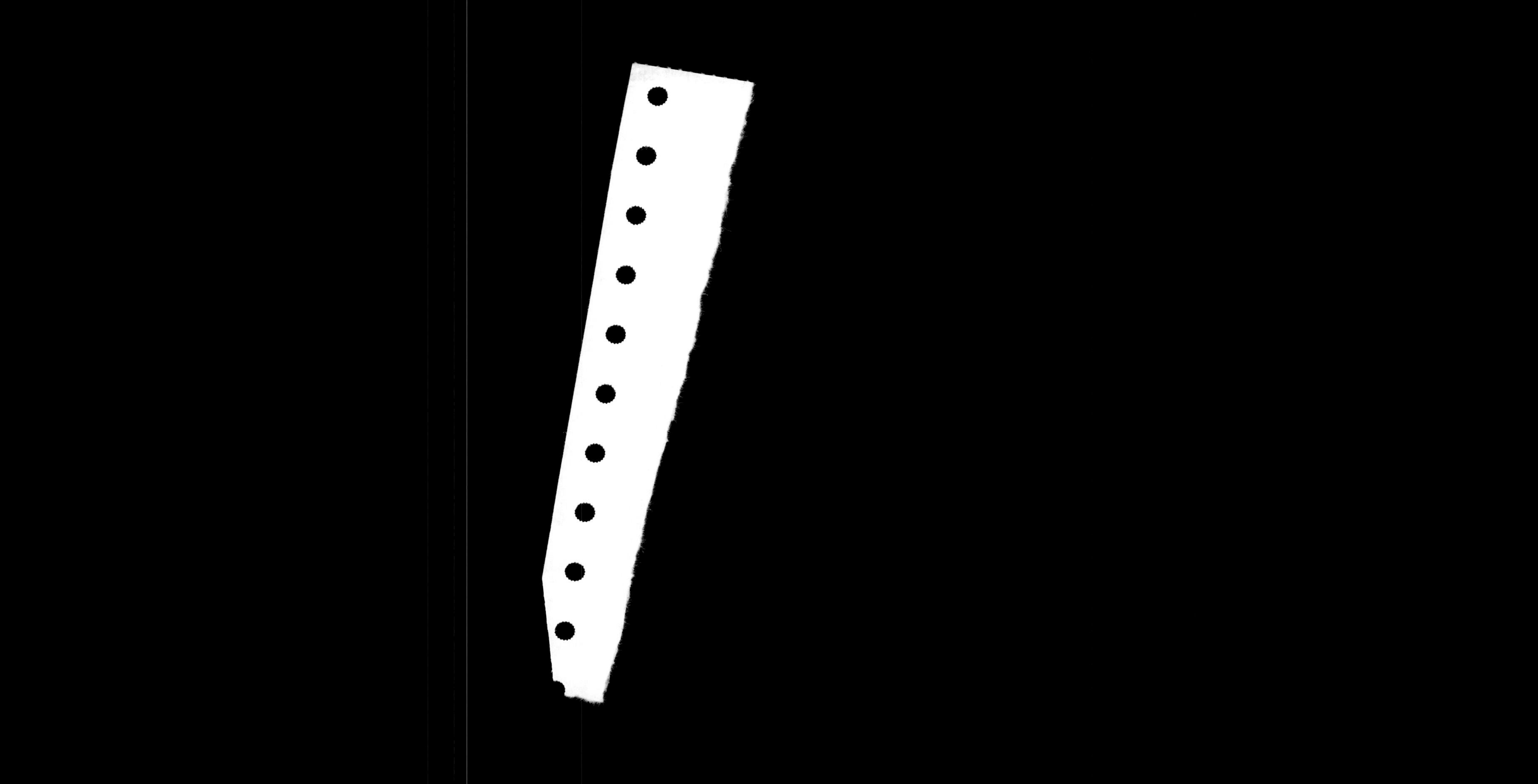

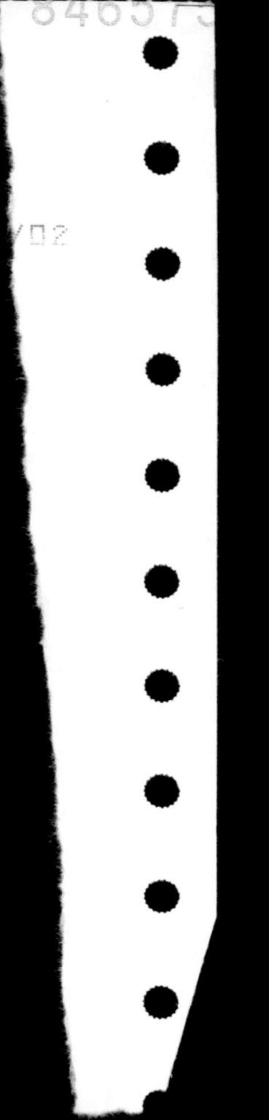

resolutely refused to go to school and Tracey protested loudly whenever Eileen left her sight. Eileen herself became reluctant to leave the house except in the company of friends and found difficulty in entering the supermarket to do her shopping. She was irritable and impatient with her children. She felt miserable and sometimes cried, especially in the evenings when she felt most alone. If she went to bed early, she knew that she would be unable to fall asleep, so she sat in front of the television set until the early hours of the morning. In fact, only television and visits from a few close friends lifted Eileen's mood. In the company of her friends, she became more animated and cheerful and more like her old self, only to become miserable again when they departed.

As with Albert, being depressed meant more to Eileen than merely feeling low in her mood. Her depression affected not only her own life but also those of her children. This is important to remember — depression can be pervasive in its effects, on the family as well as on the individual. Although Eileen had always been inclined to worry about things, she now found herself worrying unnecessarily about trivial issues. She cried and was irritable. She had difficulty falling asleep. However, there are also differences between Eileen's type of depression and Albert's. Eileen showed none of the 'biological' features like weight and appetite loss which are characteristic of endogenous depression. She suffered no delusions. Rather than waking early each morning, Eileen had most difficulty falling asleep. Her feelings of misery and despondency, unlike Albert's, were not fixed and pervasive; in the right setting, she could come out of her shell and it might then become quite difficult for others to tell that she was depressed. Her irritability and anxieties could be seen as exaggerations of 'normal' feelings, rather than being manifestly illogical or false. Most people would probably be concerned for the safety of a spouse who drove long distances, but not to the same extent as Eileen was.

Other kinds of worries may be present, but in this form of depression, they are all characteristically exaggerations of what might be considered 'normal' responses.

Being of lower than average intelligence, Robert was just beginning to discover adolescence at the age of 19. The attitudes of his friends contrasted with those of his parents, from whom he found great difficulty in separating himself. His parents were rather 'old fashioned' and Robert felt very guilty about some of his own feelings, for example, towards girls. Robert modelled himself on his closest friend with whom he often went out. This friend was tragically drowned in a swimming pool, an incident Robert witnessed. Over the next few weeks, Robert's parents noted a marked change in him. He became depressed, withdrawn and somewhat uncommunicative. He began visiting his doctor regularly, with a series of bodily complaints for which no physical cause could be found. He could feel his heart pounding, he was worried that his bowels were not as regular as they should be, he developed headaches and felt dizzy. All these complaints resolved when his depression was treated.

Symptoms like Robert's (an exaggerated preoccupation with bodily functions, which is termed hypochondriasis) and Eileen's anxiety are examples of *neurotic depression*. Here, the sufferer should be able to recognise his or her symptoms as abnormal and not take them at their face value, as someone with psychotic depression would do. In practice, this distinction between psychotic and neurotic depression is not always easy to make.

In all the case examples we have described so far, depressed mood was a characteristic feature of the overall presenting picture. However, sometimes, people who are depressed may not appear to others to be in low spirits. This may seem paradoxical until one remembers that depression entails more than feeling low. This presentation of depression without conspicuous depressed mood is called *masked depression* or *atypical depression*.

Fred, a 40-year-old man whose work involved driving a delivery van, went to see his doctor, complaining of a variety of aches and pains (especially in his neck, shoulders and back). He also said that he got excessively tired and found himself unable to do many of the things he used to, like taking his family for drives in the car at weekends. Fred himself put all his symptoms down to his pains and asked the doctor for pain killers. On closer questioning, he admitted that he was sleeping poorly and that he felt quite irritable, especially at home. He had lost his appetite and was also losing weight. With further discussion, it emerged that there was considerable tension at home. Fred had married five years previously. He and his wife had been married once before and their household included his wife's son by her first marriage and Fred's daughter by his previous marriage. Both children, now teenagers, had become rather rebellious. Although Fred and his wife considered their relationship a good one, they could not always agree when it came to controlling the children, which made matters worse. As Fred's pains and other symptoms worsened, he found himself less able to cope with the tensions and arguments at home.

This form of depression may manifest itself in other ways also; for example, some people (particularly some middle-aged women) who are caught shoplifting are found to be depressed. Here, the diagnosis of depression is reached after the discovery of features of depression in the patient's history. Pain and other bodily complaints are very common presenting features of masked depression. Where pain is the main problem, the pain itself may offer some clues as to the diagnosis. The pain may not conform to that expected from our understanding of the way the nervous system works. The intensity of the pain may vary with stress or emotional upsets.

Although such features may suggest that a person is suffering from a masked depression, it is often difficult to reach this conclusion with confidence, both for the sufferer and the doctor. The doctor has to try to ensure that the symptoms presented are not caused by any physical (that is, bodily) illness; depression may be the *result* of bodily complaints rather than their *cause*, or complaints of pain or other bodily symptoms may co-exist with physical illness, in which case both need to be investigated.

For the sufferer, the idea of 'masked depression' is often very difficult to accept. To go to the doctor with pain and to then be told that you are depressed makes it seem that the doctor does not believe that the pain is genuine. In fact, this is not so. Pain due to depression can be every bit as intense as pain due to a bodily cause and is certainly just as real. However, many people find it impossible to conceive of 'real' pain which does not have a definite physical origin. One way of attempting to understand this is to view pain as an integral part of depression. The pain is commonly 'mental' or 'psychic' pain, although for some people it is less distressing to endure such pain if it is 'translated' into bodily form. This explanation is more apparent than real, but it does allow some people to see why, when they bring their complaints of pain to their doctor, they are offered antidepressant medicines rather than pain killers. What is more, such pain often fails to respond to pain killers but may be very successfully treated with antidepressants. It is this that makes the recognition of masked depression so important.

In the elderly, depression may sometimes resemble dementia. Dementia involves the deterioration of memory, intellect and personality. It is usually progressive and, as yet, cannot be treated. It is very important to distinguish between this and depression, which can be treated as successfully in the elderly as in younger people. The depressed person's apathy, loss of interest in his surroundings and deterioration in self-care may be mistaken for dementia, giving rise to the condition known as *depressive pseudo-dementia*.

Just as depression may masquerade as some other illness or problem, the opposite can also occur, as the following history emphasises.

Joan, a nurse in her late 30s, went to her doctor because she felt tense, anxious and generally run down. The doctor knew her quite well and had in the past successfully treated her tension and anxiety with antidepressants. Joan's husband had a criminal record and her symptoms tended to get worse when he got into trouble with the police. On this occasion, however, Joan had one complaint that had never troubled her before. From time to time, she developed pains in her stomach. When the doctor examined Joan's abdomen, he could find nothing to explain these pains. He was aware (as Joan herself was) that stomach pains can be due to anxiety, and suggested to her that this was the most likely explanation for them. After some time on treatment, Joan's tension and anxiety got better but the stomach pains continued as before. It was eventually discovered that Joan had developed a stomach ulcer which caused the pains.

It was fortunate that Joan's ulcer was discovered before its effects had been particularly damaging. Joan's experience serves as a cautionary tale, reminding us that what appears to be depression *may* sometimes be the first sign of a physical illness, which needs proper investigation and treatment in its own right. In some ways, Joan had been quite lucky — she had developed a new symptom that was not typical of those found in depression. Opinions differ about how commonly physical illnesses show themselves as depression, but the main point is that it *does* happen — this is well recognised. This is one reason why people who go to their doctor complaining of feeling depressed will sometimes be asked to have blood tests and other investigations. However, it remains true that the vast majority of people who have no complaints beyond those we described earlier in this chapter are suffering from depression rather than some other problem or illness.

As we shall see, there are a variety of ways in which depression might be treated or managed and different treatments suit particular types of depression. What helps one type of depression may even make another type worse. Depression as a whole has a multitude of causes but certain causative factors are more common in some types of depression than in others. So deciding what type of depression a person suffers goes some way towards suggesting appropriate treatments and providing more clues about the way that individual may have become depressed. Unfortunately, the classification of depression into different types is an area of considerable complexity and even experts cannot always agree about it. There are a number of different ways of classifying depression, none of which is so successful as to supersede all the others. The types of depression we have described in this chapter do not all fit into the same classification, but have been chosen because they are talked about relatively often.

We have used several different syndromes to review the main presenting features of depression. Some of these features are exceedingly common in the general population: at any one time, one in every five adults will admit to having some of the symptoms already described. By contrast, the 'syndromes' of depression are much less common: at any given time, between 0.5 per cent and 5 per cent of the adult population will be suffering severe depression, like Albert's.

Some people recover from depression and never suffer from it again. Others are less fortunate and may have recurrent episodes of depression. In general, once a person has suffered one depressive episode, especially a severe one, he or she stands a greater than average risk of having further episodes. Some people who have recurrent bouts of 'endogenous' depression may also go on to have episodes of mania. In simple terms, this can be viewed as the opposite of depression — the manic person is extremely overactive, intrusive in manner and expansive in gesture and thought. His or her elation is often infectious, making others laugh too. At first, this change in mental state may be regarded as positive and desirable, but quickly becomes uncontrollable and then requires urgent treatment. Someone who is manic may also have delusions and may experience hallucinations (for example, hearing voices when no one is speaking). This picture of bouts of depression plus bouts of mania is called *manic depressive psychosis* or *bipolar affective disorder*.

By studying the patterns of depression in people who have recurrent episodes, it is possible to suggest factors which may be especially important in predicting such a relapsing picture. For example, someone who has had episodes of mania as well as bouts of depression is more likely to suffer episodes of depression in the future than is a person who has never been manic. There is also some evidence that people with the 'endogenous' pattern of depression are more likely to return to their 'normal' selves after treatment than those with some types of neurotic depression. However, all such prediction is based on the laws of chance and probability, and is thus of limited use to the individual sufferer — the fact that there is, say, only a one in twenty chance that a particular unwanted event may occur offers little consolation if we happen to suffer that event. For individual sufferers, the pattern of their depression is likely to become clear over time. For instance, after several episodes of depression, some people come to recognise that their depression always begins with the same features. This is important because early recognition of the problem allows it to be dealt with before it becomes severe.

It is usual for episodes of depression to be limited in time — recovery is the general rule. For a small percentage of sufferers, the depression may continue for many years. For some of these people, observation of their complaints over time eventually leads to the conclusion that they were not suffering from depression as such. Others do have depression but this proves resistant to treatment.

When does depression become an illness? When should someone who has symptoms of depression be considered to suffer from a 'depressive illness'? There is no single correct answer to these questions. Broadly speaking, depression is unlikely to be considered an illness unless it becomes so intrusive that it interferes significantly with the life of the person experiencing it or with the lives of those around him or her. Often, this is the point at which a person will choose to seek help, either from a doctor or from someone else. However, this is not always so — individuals and families vary considerably in their tolerance of depression and other discomfort. Some people who are severely depressed do not seek help, while others will try to find help when their discomfort is minimal. It is not only the depressed person who suffers; sometimes, family and friends can be very severely affected, as some of our case histories have suggested.

Even when depression is severe, it may not be regarded as an illness. During grief, for example, the bereaved will possibly suffer most of the symptoms of depression we have described. Far from seeing grief during bereavement as an illness, it is commonly regarded as an important process through which people must go, however painful it might be to them. Symptoms usually associated with depressive illness are, in the context of bereavement, considered quite normal. Hence a 'depressive illness' represents more than the experience of the symptoms of depression, however severe they might be.

Our example of bereavement may be taken further. Death has different meanings in different cultures and the effects of bereavement will similarly be influenced by its social and cultural context. In some societies, grief is very public; in others, the bereaved are expected to grieve privately and present a dignified façade. Every society sanctions its particular form of bereavement. Although customs may differ markedly from one society to another, while we are able to grieve in the manner expected of us, few if any of our relatives or friends would regard us as 'ill'. Bereavement thus has a social dimension, and a person's grief can only be adequately understood in its social and cultural context. The same applies to depression. It is permissible to express feelings of hopelessness and misery in some societies but not in others. This is likely to influence the ways in which depression may manifest itself. Our account of depression, above, relates to Western societies, especially to countries like Britain and the United States.

Further consideration of the social context of health and illness, though fascinating, is complex and beyond the scope of this book. One final point is worth making, about the role of the doctor. We tend to go to the doctor to get treatment for 'illnesses'. It is the doctor who, in a sense, gives us permission to be ill by giving our problems a label (or diagnosis), writing the sick note for our employers and so on. Many people see their doctor as someone who only deals with 'illness' and has to define his patients' problems in such terms before being able to help. This is not true, because some of the people doctors treat are very healthy (like pregnant mothers). Nevertheless, the idea persists that one visits the doctor and comes away with an illness. This may be one reason why many people who become depressed are now turning for help to therapists other than their doctors.

CHAPTER TWO

Conventional Methods of Treatment

If someone who is depressed seeks help from a doctor, what should he or she expect? Before considering some of the options doctors may have available to help those with depression, several general points deserve emphasis.

First, why *treat* depression? If, as we learnt in the last chapter, many episodes of depression are self-limiting and likely to end in recovery, why bother with any intervention? To many of those people who have themselves received treatment for depression, the answer to this question may seem obvious but it is nonetheless worth restating. Depression may be a source of great discomfort and distress not only to sufferers but also to their loved ones. Successful treatment minimises this. If it is allowed to become severe, untreated depression is also dangerous because of the significant risk of suicide (not all episodes of depression progress to become severe, but it is often difficult to predict how a particular episode will develop, especially when the individual has never previously experienced depression). It is with this knowledge that the benefits and costs of treatment must be weighed. *All* treatments and interventions, no matter how innocuous they may seem, have costs as well as benefits. Although the costs, or hazards, of treatment are most commonly associated in the public eye with drugs and their side-effects, other treatments can also be detrimental. For example, encouraging someone who is severely depressed to explore the basis for his or her current feelings may exacerbate ideas of guilt and worthlessness and worsen the depression. Persisting with any type of ineffectual treatment is hazardous since this runs the risk of the depression worsening. Thus a treatment which may in itself be harmless can have harmful effects through continuing use.

While most treatments are designed to have specific effects, without exception they also have what are called *placebo* effects. A placebo is any treatment which, although without any known specific effect on the condition being treated, produces a change (either improvement or deterioration) in an individual's symptoms or illness. In the pre-scientific era, physicians and healers understood such effects very well because the vast majority of their remedies probably were placebos, without any direct effects on the individual's illness. This led to the idea that healers should 'treat as many patients with the new remedies while they still have the power to heal'. Such effects are not imaginary — they are very real and can be very powerful.

The placebo effect is important in depression. Even if very strict criteria are used to decide whether a person is depressed or not, a significant proportion of any group of depressed people will respond to treatment with a placebo. It follows that, in order to establish any particular treatment as specifically effective for depression, it is not enough to offer the evidence of individual cases which have shown good response to this particular treatment, as this might well represent a placebo response. Nevertheless, most treatments begin in this way — a few successes suggest that the treatment concerned is worthy of closer scrutiny and evaluation. To be convincing, the results of any treatment need to be compared with those obtained using placebos. This approach is relatively easy to adopt when studying the effects of treatment with drugs but becomes much more difficult with other therapies, particularly those which are 'tailor made' for each individual sufferer. Most of the treatments to be discussed in this chapter have been investigated and validated in this way. We shall return to the placebo response again in the next chapter.

If you go to a doctor with depression, at least two conditions need to be met before you are likely to be offered any treatment. First, the doctor will want to satisfy himself that you are indeed depressed. Amongst other things, he will ask you about the features of depression which we have already described. The second condition of treatment is that you and the doctor agree that the depression is severe enough to make treatment not only appropriate but also necessary.

The final general point to stress is that, for the individual with depression, there is seldom one particular treatment which completely overshadows all others in its potential benefits. A number of different therapies may stand an equal chance of success. What is more, these therapeutic options are not necessarily incompatible; two types of treatment used together may in some instances be more effective than either used alone. Only when depression is severe does the range of effective treatments become somewhat narrower. Because two therapists offer different treatments does not mean that one of these treatments is necessarily 'wrong' or ineffective. The choice of treatment or treatments will depend both on the needs of the depressed individual and on the skills of the therapist. The depressed person will want a treatment which has a good chance of success but whose hazards are not intolerable. The therapist is likely to choose a certain therapy (or set of therapies) whose use he understands and is skilled at applying. For someone who has recurrent episodes of depression, it may be appropriate to choose a treatment which has succeeded in helping him in the past.

Treatment with drugs

The form of treatment which the public most commonly associates with doctors is the use of medicines or drugs. Drugs which are intended to have a specific effect in treating depression are, not surprisingly, called antidepressants. Until quite recently, the commonly used antidepressants all belonged to one of two groups of drug: they were either tricyclic antidepressants or monoamine oxidase inhibitors. Now, increasing use is being made of so-called 'new generation' antidepressants.

The tricyclic antidepressants are so named because they all share the same basic chemical 'skeleton'. Tricyclics are often the drugs of first choice in treating depression; they are particularly helpful in those depressions in which biological features are evident (for example, psychotic or so-called endogenous types of depression), but are also often effective in other types of depression. The current British National Formulary (which lists all drugs available to prescribers in Britain) contains ten different tricyclic antidepressants. All have been shown to be more effective than placebos in treating depression, and the choice of one particular drug in preference to the others depends on their different side-effects and on the doctor's customary practice. Although the tricyclics are more liable than the 'new generation' drugs to produce side-effects, they are still preferred by many doctors because their efficacy has been better established because they have been in use for longer periods than the newer drugs.

Like most other antidepressants, the tricyclics are only effective in treating depression if taken regularly, in adequate dosage, for at least two weeks. Taking the odd antidepressant tablet or capsule when one feels low is worse than useless; taking the drugs for a few days then stopping is also not helpful, because they will not have had an adequate chance to work and the two-week 'countdown' must start afresh when the treatment is resumed.

Unfortunately, although there is this lag period before the therapeutic effects may be felt, the side-effects of the drug, when they occur, tend to start immediately. One side-effect that is sometimes desirable is sedation — some tricyclics cause drowsiness. This can be very helpful to those depressed people who have experienced sleep difficulties or who are very agitated. Here, the drug may be given as a single dose at night. Some tricyclics are more sedative than others; if neither agitation nor lack of sleep are problems; it is often preferable to use a less sedative drug. Other relatively common side-effects include dry mouth, blurring of vision, sweating, difficulty in passing urine and constipation. In the elderly, tricyclics (like almost all other drugs) may sometimes produce confusion. It is important to realise that such complaints are not always due to the drugs but may be part of the depression itself — it is sometimes difficult to distinguish between these. Other unwanted effects of these drugs are less common; like all other side-effects, these are best seen in the context of the particular individual having the treatment and our advice to anyone worried about such effects is to discuss them further with the doctor who prescribed the drug.

Not everyone experiences side-effects. Some people have none, while others appear to be exquisitely sensitive to any drug they take. As we have already stressed, side-effects must be weighed up against the likely benefits of the treatment and the potential hazards of the continuing depression. One should not expect taking any medicine to be as harmless as eating chocolates. The same principle applies to other effective therapies. Any side-effects tend to be at their worst at the start of treatment, often subsiding after a few days. It is thus especially important to persevere with them for more than a day or two.

Two other points regarding adverse effects are worth stressing. Some drugs produce side-effects that are irreversible — they do not go away. This does not apply to the antidepressants, the adverse effects of which all disappear when you stop taking the drug. Also, some drugs like Valium (see below) are addictive, and once one has taken them regularly for a while it becomes very difficult to stop. Antidepressants do not produce addiction to this extent, even when they are taken for long periods of time.

Like other drugs, tricyclics are available in different strengths. Taking six capsules or tablets at night does not usually mean that this is a very large dose, but merely that the amount of drug in each tablet is relatively small. This allows the dose of the drug to be changed much more flexibly to suit individual needs and sensitivity. Another point which often baffles people about their prescriptions is the different names given to the same drug. All drugs have a 'generic' name which describes their chemical structure. The same drug may be manufactured by different drug companies, each of which will give the drug their own 'brand' name; thus Domical, Elavil, Lentizol, Saroten or Tryptizol (brand names) are all preparations available in Britain of the common tricyclic, amitriptyline (generic name), but manufactured by different companies. To further complicate this picture, drugs sold in different countries may have different 'brand' names, although they are known everywhere by the same generic name.

Monoamine oxidase inhibitors (or MAOI's) interfere with the action of a particular enzyme called monoamine oxidase, which occurs not only in the brain but also in other parts of the body (we shall touch on the possible relevance of this enzyme to our understanding of depression in Chapter Nine). The discovery of the MAOI's is a story of pharmacological serendipity. It was observed that patients who had tuberculosis became rather euphoric when treated with one particular anti-tuberculous drug called iproniazid. This chance observation led pharmacologists to make a number of drugs like iproniazid which were then tested for their antidepressant effects. Among these were the first MAOI's. This is by no means an unusual story — many major therapeutic breakthroughs have started with chance or anecdotal observations. This is worth remembering when we come to discuss the alternative therapies in Chapter Three.

The MAOI's have been shown to be particularly effective in treating people with atypical depression or depression without biological features, though some doctors also advocate their use in other forms of depression. The side-effects of these drugs are similar to those described above for the tricyclics, but may also include headaches or dizziness. Like others antidepressants, the side-effects of the MAOI's cease when the drug is stopped, and the drugs themselves are not addictive. However, there is one potentially hazardous side-effect called the 'cheese reaction', and because of this the MAOI's are not used by most doctors as frequently as are the other antidepressants. To understand the cheese reaction, we need to consider how monoamine oxidase works in the body: it breaks down monoamines, which are a class of chemical messenger. Amongst their many functions, monoamines are involved in the regulation of blood pressure — an increase in monoamines in the blood causes a rise in blood pressure. Certain foods contain monoamines which are absorbed in the gut and released into the body. These monoamines could precipitate a considerable rise in blood pressure, but for the action of monoamine oxidase, which normally breaks down the ingested monoamines, rendering them harmless. If monoamine oxidase is prevented from acting by an MAOI, the monoamines are not broken down and a dramatic rise in blood pressure (called a hypertensive crisis) may result. This is usually heralded by a severe headache and requires urgent medical attention. For this reason, people taking MAOI's have to follow the 'MAOI diet', avoiding foods which contain significant amounts of monoamines, such as cheese, pickled herrings, broad bean pods, meat or yeast extracts (like Oxo, Bovril and Marmite) and some other products like chianti wine. Certain medicines (including some available over the counter without a prescription) also have a similar effect, so people taking MAOI's must be cautious about other medicines they take. Doctors will often give their patients on this treatment a special 'MAOI Treatment Card' to remind them of the precautions they need to take.

As the standard MAOI's and tricyclic antidepressants have been available for some years, their use and efficacy are well understood. In this respect, the long-established drugs have a considerable advantage over newer antidepressants, even though the latter are always put through rigorous clinical trials before they become available for general use. Compared with the standard antidepressants, none of the new drugs has been shown to be any more effective in treating depression, and they are more expensive. For all these reasons, many doctors use the older tricyclics in preference to the newer antidepressants whenever possible. However, the newer drugs are less likely to produce unwanted side-effects and are thus particularly useful when the side-effects of the tricyclics might prove especially troublesome.

Antidepressants are not only used to treat specific episodes of depression. When someone has been severely depressed, there is a significant risk of relapse into further depression if the treatment is stopped too soon. In such instances, treatment is often continued for some months after the person has recovered, to minimise this risk. Longer-term treatment with antidepressants is sometimes recommended for some people who are prone to recurrent episodes of depression; even if such treatment (which is called *prophylactic*) does not entirely prevent further episodes of depression, it usually lessens their severity. Another drug used in this way, to reduce the chances of further depressive episodes, is lithium — one of the oldest established drugs in psychiatry, having been used successfully since the late 1940s. It was originally used to treat mania and is still widely prescribed for the prophylaxis of manic depressive disorder. Like the other drugs described above, lithium can only be effective if taken regularly in adequate doses. Because it may, in some instances, cause gradual changes in the functioning of the kidneys or thyroid gland, regular blood tests are done to monitor its effects. When administered properly in this way, lithium is not only effective but can also be used safely.

In the past, extensive use was made of diazepam (Valium) and related drugs belonging to the class of drugs called benzodiazepines. Although these are not specifically antidepressants, their calming effects were found useful in treating the anxiety and agitation which often accompanies depression. More recently, it has become apparent that these drugs can be very addictive when used continually for periods longer than a few weeks. After long-term use, it sometimes proves difficult to stop taking them because the body becomes dependent on them. 'Withdrawal effects' from such drugs are common, especially if they are discontinued abruptly. Such effects are not dissimilar from the anxiety the drug was intended to treat. This capacity of the benzodiazepines to produce dependence is one reason why doctors have become much more cautious in prescribing them, especially for courses of treatment lasting longer than a couple of weeks.

Psychotherapy

Even when depression becomes quite incapacitating, treatment with drugs is not necessarily useful or even appropriate.

Mary was a 47-year-old housewife, whose husband Bill confessed to her that he had had a brief affair with a female colleague at work. Bill felt considerable remorse over this and tried hard to make amends. Mary seemed very understanding about it all but after some months began to complain of tiredness, dizziness and headaches. Her symptoms gradually worsened, but despite repeated visits to her own doctor no physical cause for her complaints could be discovered. Bill asked the doctor to refer Mary to a specialist physician at the hospital, and took time off from work to accompany her to her appointments. After several visits to the specialists, the cause of Mary's problems seemed no clearer and she had now also begun to lose weight. Her doctor noticed that she looked increasingly miserable whenever she attended his surgery; she admitted to him that the mornings were especially difficult for her and that she sometimes cried then, but could offer no reason for doing so. Suspecting that Mary's symptoms were due to depression, the doctor wanted to refer her to a psychiatrist. Both Mary and Bill were initially opposed to this and Bill, believing that Mary was suffering from some serious physical illness as yet undiagnosed, insisted that Mary be referred to another specialist physician for a second opinion. With the help of the specialist, Mary's doctor finally persuaded her to seek psychiatric help. It emerged that the relationship between Mary and Bill, although very warm when they first married, changed after the birth of their son, now 17 years old. He had been a sickly child and, until recently, had suffered quite severely from asthma. Mary and Bill devoted all their energy to keeping their son well and advancing his schooling. He was now in good health and planning to leave home in a few weeks' time to go to university.

When changes happen within a family, they commonly affect everyone in the family. For Bill and Mary, being husband and wife took second place to being parents. Mary had devoted herself for years to being a mother, a particularly important role while her son was unwell but one which she would effectively lose when he left home. Bill's brief affair had threatened Mary's role as a partner much more than either of them could admit and Mary's apparently understanding response to the affair hid a great deal of turmoil and uncertainty. All this remained unresolved, as Mary and Bill had never been accustomed to 'talking things through'. Mary's illness drew Bill closer to her and gave him the opportunity to demonstrate how much he cared for her, making sure that she received medical attention and so on. Sadly, couples like this sometimes go from one practitioner to another in search of a more palatable solution to their distress. Here, treating Mary with any form of medicine would reinforce the idea that Mary was 'ill' and, with it, the uncomfortable compromise she and Bill had reached in their relationship. A much more appropriate approach is to talk to Mary, either individually or together with her husband, to help them relinquish her role as an 'ill person' and to enjoy her roles as an individual and as a partner.

Such treatment would be one example of psychotherapy. This literally means *any* treatment applied to a mental, or 'psychic' disorder. However, the term is commonly used to denote any treatments that use 'psychological' means. Even in this more restricted sense, psychotherapy covers a wide variety of approaches. At one extreme, anyone who consoles a distraught friend is practising psychotherapy. There are people, without any recognised or specific training, who advertise themselves as psychotherapists; such 'therapists' are best avoided. There are, however, some more specific kinds of psychotherapy which may be useful to someone who is depressed.

Supportive psychotherapy should be one component of all treatments for depression. This may involve no more than the therapist listening to the depressed person's problems, advising about symptoms and helping the individual to recognise how his depression came about. This alone is often sufficient help for the depressed person. Recent research has shown that this approach can be just as effective as medications in treating the kinds of depression seen by doctors in general practice. Other research has revealed that some people who visit their general practitioner with depression may benefit from help from a social worker, particularly when they lack emotional support and have social problems needing practical assistance.

Sometimes, it is sufficient for the therapist to give the depressed person 'permission' to be depressed.

Arthur was a life-long bachelor, a solitary man who, since his retirement, spent most of his time reading books from his local library and watching television. He was very fond of his pet dog, whom he used to take for daily walks in a nearby park. When eventually the dog died (of 'old age'), Arthur became miserable and his interest in his books declined. He was angry at the suggestion of his neighbour that all would be well again if he got himself another dog. He eventually visited his doctor because he was unable to sleep well at night and always felt exhausted.

Had Arthur lost a close relative rather than a pet, he would have been able to accept his feelings and probably not sought his doctor's help. However, mourning the loss of a pet seemed rather foolish. Arthur was considerably relieved when the doctor reflected that his dog had been very important to him and that his grief was understandable and legitimate. He went away without any medicines.

All supportive psychotherapy avoids addressing the depressed person's 'inner world'. By contrast, this is the chief focus for the different types of dynamic (or interpretative) psychotherapy. There are many different schools of dynamic psychotherapy, all aimed at helping the individual to gain better understanding of his inner feelings. The dynamic psychotherapies are commonly considered to have originated with the work of Sigmund Freud, who developed psychoanalysis. Since Freud's time, other schools have developed, including Jung's analytic psychology, Adler's individual psychology and numerous others. Each school has its own theories and techniques, in which practitioners generally have to undergo a lengthy period of training. Some psychiatrists use a psychotherapeutic approach in their treatment, but this is often eclectic in nature rather than being firmly rooted in one particular psychotherapeutic school. Psychologists, social workers and general practitioners may also adopt such an approach. In Britain, it is possible to obtain dynamic psychotherapy on the National Health Service, but this is not widely available.

Psychotherapy is not always aimed at the individual. In Mary's case, which we mentioned earlier, it was suggested that she and Bill together should have some marital therapy. Sometimes, a whole family is recommended to come for therapy, even when there appears to be only one person in the family who has 'the problem'. Sometimes, group therapy is suggested, in which a number of people join together in trying to work out their difficulties with the help of one or more therapists. If it is suggested to any of us that we have psychotherapy, the particular form of therapy will depend on the therapist's assessment of our individual needs and how these could best be met.

The place of the dynamic psychotherapies in the treatment of depression remains controversial. There are some who believe that all formal psychotherapy is merely an expensive placebo, while others recommend its use to treat all types of depression. One reason for this lack of agreement has been the difficulty in evaluating the effects of psychotherapy. As we mentioned before, the methods used to decide whether drug treatments are effective do not lend themselves to the assessment of psychotherapy. Until recently, attempts to devise other methods appropriate to psychotherapy have proved largely unsuccessful, but there are now signs that this is beginning to change.

Antidepressants and psychotherapy tend to have diffferent effects on the symptoms of depression; antidepressants (especially the tricyclics) are very effective in treating biological symptoms, while psychotherapy is more helpful in dealing with the 'psychic' symptoms. There is some evidence that, for some kinds of depression, the two treatments together are more effective than each alone. Most doctors would probably argue that dynamic psychotherapy has little place in the early stages of a depressive episode, especially if it is severe. However, once the immediate symptoms of depression have been successfully treated, psychotherapy may be helpful to address some of the possible factors contributing to the depression.

Janet became depressed at the end of her pregnancy. She had responded to some extent to antidepressants and would not have struck the casual observer as any longer depressed. In herself, though, she felt somehow empty, as though she had lost part of her former self. She was an intelligent, articulate woman, who had never achieved her full potential. She commented that she was lucky to have scraped through her university degree course, but had not used her degree, choosing instead to do clerical work until she became pregnant. She was an only child whose parents divorced when she was 6 years old. Her mother remarried but her stepfather, like her father, was a rather cold and distant man whom she felt she had never got to know well. She married a man thirty years older than herself. The pregnancy was unplanned — they were undecided whether or not to have any children. Janet was initially very enthusiastic about having a child, but her husband viewed the prospect of becoming a father at his age with some concern. After the birth, Janet's husband decided for himself that anything to do with the child's upbringing should be his wife's responsibility.

Pregnancy and the post-natal period are times when women are particularly vulnerable to depression (see Chapter Nine). However, Janet's depression involved more than the biological changes associated with childbirth. When she was first married, her relationship with her husband was more like that between daughter and father than a partnership of equals; her husband became for her the caring father she felt she had previously lacked. This relationship between Janet and her husband was profoundly affected by the birth of their child. Although Janet undoubtedly benefited from the antidepressants she took at the start of her depressive episode, they still left her feeling 'lost' and different from her former self. Psychotherapy helped her to link her present feelings of being unloved and abandoned with similar feelings she had had about her own father and step-father.

Psychotherapy of this kind is not a treatment to embark upon lightly. Some people may view psychotherapy as a soft option — a pleasurable experience, of which they may be the passive recipients, and which leaves them feeling better. In fact, the person undergoing therapy must have a great deal of commitment and, during the course of the therapy, should expect to do 'emotional work' which may be very distressing and painful. This is one reason why someone who is referred to a psychotherapist will usually be offered a period of assessment (one or a few sessions) to decide whether this form of treatment would be suitable and potentially beneficial.

One other type of psychotherapy which deserves specific mention is cognitive therapy. Based on the cognitive theory of depression (see Chapter Nine), cognitive therapy aims to make the individual aware of the depressive and negative thoughts which are prominent in depression.

Brian was admitted to hospital after an overdose of a friend's tablets. At work, he had been reprimanded by his boss for being careless in completing a task. He took this criticism badly and was still miserable when he got home that evening. He tried to telephone his girlfriend to tell her what had happened. When he first tried to phone her, there was no answer. He told himself she was not yet back from work. When he tried again a little later, the phone was engaged. He made several more attempts to phone, but her line was continually engaged. When he looked back on this later, Brian could not understand why he felt so badly at that time, but, apparently on impulse, he took some of his flatmate's tablets he found in the bathroom.

Talking to Brian after his admission to hospital, it became clear that he went through periods when the smallest setback seemed to him like a disaster of enormous proportions. He saw everything in very negative terms. When he talked over with the therapist what happened on the evening of his overdose, Brian realised that he had the thought in his mind at that time that his girlfriend had deliberately left her phone off the hook because she did not want to talk to him. Following his trivial setback at work, the whole world began to look bleak. With the therapist's help, Brian was able to look at this event more objectively, suggesting a few more plausible explanations for the phone being engaged — this process is called 'cognitive restructuring' (changing the structure, or connotation, of thoughts). In effect, Brian was helped to test his thoughts about this event against the reality of the situation, and having done this, he was able to see what happened in a different light. With further practice, Brian became able to recognise many of the other occasions when he developed such negative thoughts. Not only did he become more aware of the thoughts themselves, but he was able to do something about these thoughts by himself, using the techniques he had been taught.

Cognitive therapy is being used increasingly in the treatment of depression, particularly by psychologists but also by psychiatrists and other doctors who have trained in its use. Research has established its efficacy, although there remain unanswered questions about its use — for example, do some types of depression respond more favourably to cognitive therapy than others?

In Britain, most general practitioners have direct access to, or themselves undertake, all the therapies we have so far considered. Two other treatments should be mentioned for the sake of completeness, both of which are usually prescribed not by general practitioners but by psychiatric specialists. Electroconvulsive therapy (ECT) is commonly recommended in severe depression to alleviate marked distress, or when other treatments have failed or are inappropriate. There is no doubt that ECT is an effective treatment for depression, but the controversy surrounding its use is beyond the scope of this book. The same applies to psychosurgery — brain surgery for mental illness. This is infrequently recommended to people who continue to suffer from long-standing depression which has not responded to any other treatment.

CHAPTER THREE

Alternative and Non-medical Treatments: An Introduction

President Nixon's visit to China in 1972 initiated a new phase in East–West relations. He and his enormous entourage were shown many things which had previously attracted little attention in the West, and brought back seemingly incredible reports of patients being treated with acupuncture. Since then there has been a vast increase in interest in all forms of alternative medicine, indeed a recent study in Britain showed that alternative health care is now growing at an annual rate of 11 per cent. Why should this be, at a time when scientific medicine is advancing so rapidly?

Alternative approaches to treatment have been around for a long time. Even acupuncture is by no means a new import to the West; there have been a few acupuncturists working in Europe since the early part of the nineteenth century, and perhaps even earlier. Similarly, herbal medicine and manipulation have been available for hundreds of years. The heyday of homoeopathy in both Europe and the United States was in the last half of the nineteenth century. Many had thought that the rise of scientific rationalism would bury these therapeutic approaches for good.

There are undoubtedly many reasons for this. The rate of progress in medical research is staggering — it is estimated that the sum total of all medical knowledge is now doubling every seven years. Although we know ever more about the causes and the treatment of disease, for individual sufferers progress will never seem sufficiently rapid until we can restore and maintain their health permanently. So, in the meantime, people will go elsewhere to try to find treatment and cures, even when these treatments may not have been scientifically proven to work.

Although we are becoming so good at dealing with physical disease, all illnesses have both physical and mental components. It might often seem that we are neglecting the mental side of illness. Most doctors have always been acutely aware of the importance of dealing with the whole person, but the twin constraints of time and money often make this difficult. It is in this area that alternative practitioners score. Most will spend a good deal of time with the client, and this in itself will often do as much if not more than any form of therapy which they administer.

This leads us to a most important issue — the placebo response, which we have already mentioned in Chapter Two. There is a considerable scientific literature on what happens during a placebo reaction. Some years ago it was shown that at least some placebo reactions are associated with the release from the brain of a particular set of chemicals called endorphins. It has been shown possible to block one type of placebo reaction with a drug called naloxone which interferes with some of the actions of endorphins. This means that *any* type of treatment can have a physical effect on the body. Whatever the ultimate causes of the placebo response, it is very clear that it can be immensely powerful. There is good evidence that placebo treatments — for instance, administering dummy tablets — can have profound effects on the body, changing the secretion of various hormones, and even altering some elements of the immune system. More importantly still, many forms of pain and psychological distress can be abolished.

The existence of the placebo response is regarded as crucial when trying to evaluate scientifically any form of treatment, be it a drug for depression or a homoeopathic remedy. As we mentioned previously, when doing a trial of a new drug it is often compared with a dummy tablet, and the result of the trial is expressed as the difference between the new drug and the dummy. When investigating alternative therapies, such an approach may not be valid, and it has led to major problems in conducting trials of this form of therapy. It must be pointed out that the same sort of problems apply to psychotherapy. This is a relatively accepted form of treatment but it is hard to apply normal scientific tests to prove that it works.

Of course, as far as the individual is concerned, that a treatment works is more important than how it does so. Every form of treatment has its failures as well as its successes, but careful observation of several therapies over a period of some years now has shown that many of them do indeed seem to be effective. It must be stressed that these are primarily personal observations, and with virtually all the medical alternatives we still lack positive scientific evidence that they work. In most cases the studies have just not been done and we have had to rely on our personal observations and impressions. It will be interesting to see what science discovers about these things in the future.

It is the belief of the authors that the alternatives to conventional medical treatment should all be expected to produce research to back their claims in the same way that medical scientists have to prove that a treatment works, and what the cost of the treatment is in terms of side-effects or other unwanted reactions. This will not be easy but the first steps are being taken, with the co-operation of doctors and alternative therapists.

One of the major difficulties in investigating alternative medicine is one that we shall return to several times. The doctor and the alternative practitioner look at the client in totally different ways. The doctor looks at the person as a highly sophisticated machine; disease is an imbalance somewhere in that machine. Even if the disease has been caused by some social stress, it is still this machine that goes wrong. We shall learn that there are many types of alternative medicine, each with its own techniques and beliefs, but they all share the idea that there is something more to people than being a machine. For them there is certainly a spirit and a soul, and many also believe in different forms of body energy. They feel that it is necessary to minister to all of these, not just to the physical body. All the alternative therapies stress the importance of the will to get better. For many of them, their therapies are primarily designed to put the patient in a position where he heals himself. With such different points of view, it may seem impossible to reconcile the two. We are optimistic. We think it is quite possible for the two camps to look at each and work together. We have spent some time on this because these different points of view explain why there is such a difference between a visit to the doctor or to the alternative practitioner. Earlier on we discussed the way in which depression is classified medically. The whole point of doing this classification is so that we can make predictions concerning treatment and outcome. Having gone through this process, the doctor decides on a treatment based on his experience of dealing with people who have also had this diagnosis. On the other hand, the alternative practitioner sets out to deal with the whole person. So although you might go to, say, a homoeopath, complaining of depression, he would set about treating a number of factors which are specific to you as an individual. Different people who might seem to have the same form of depression would receive quite different treatments.

This second approach can be very appealing to some folk. Perhaps the desire to have this tailor-made form of treatment reflects a more general social trend. People like to be seen as individuals. Doctors often do in fact try to use a similar approach themselves, but it has never been publicised in the same way. From what we know about placebos, it is clear that this way of approaching patients will have a strong placebo effect, whatever else the treatment may or may not do.

There are also other reasons why people are going to alternative therapists. The treatments are for the most part relatively harmless, although harm may occur if a person is treated inappropriately. There have undoubtedly been some cases of physical damage caused particularly by acupuncture and chiropractice, but there have been few of these, and after all, conventional medicine also causes a good many problems, primarily from the unwanted effects of drugs.

In the past, many doctors were extremely unhappy about the use of alternative medicine. Cynics have said that this was because doctors were afraid of losing their monopoly on health care, but this is not the main reason. The principal concern of doctors is to see their patients get better. There have been two worrying problems. The first is that the use of a non-medical treatment may mask or cause the failure to notice some more serious underlying disease. This is very uncommon, but the authors know one patient to whom this very thing happened. The second is the inappropriate use of a therapy. Nobody would use just a Band Aid to treat a gunshot wound, and yet we have seen people with serious disease who have been treated unsuccessfully with a single type of alternative therapy, when conventional medicine had curative treatment to offer. It is for these reasons that we must reiterate that if you or a member of your family decides to opt for alternative medical treatment of any form, then this must be with the knowledge and consent of your own physician. Doctors are now themselves becoming very interested in the treatment alternatives and will for the most part be supportive of the idea. If they feel that such a form of treatment is not appropriate they will usually tell you why. It is also important that if you do go for alternative treatment you can and indeed should continue with your conventional medical treatment until the doctor thinks it safe and reasonable to stop.

Finally, if you do decide to consult an alternative practitioner, do first make sure that he or she is properly trained. We shall go into this in more detail in later chapters. This leads us to the vexed question of whether you should only consult a medically qualified alternative practitioner. Perhaps in an ideal world all therapists should be medically qualified as well. However, many doctors find it difficult to learn alternative medical techniques. Furthermore, there will not be enough of them for the foreseeable future to deal with the ever-rising demand. So for now, we feel that it is a reasonable compromise to say that alternative treatment should only be done under medical supervision.

There are well over a hundred forms of alternative treatment and it would not be possible to discuss all of them and do them all justice. There are a number of excellent books available which deal with the finer points of these therapies. What we present here is the result of several years spent investigating a small number of therapies in detail. This was not a formal scientific evaluation, it was rather the result of a good deal of time spent studying the techniques in question and watching practitioners at work. It is worth bearing in mind that many medical discoveries were made in just this way. An anecdotal report was followed by a formal investigation and then attempts were made to understand the basis of what had been observed. This is an exciting time, we are seeing this whole age-old procedure in action. Largely because of the different way in which alternative practitioners look at people, only a small number of the patients we saw treated had actually had formal medical diagnoses attached to them. In the next stage, it will be interesting to see how people get on with alternative therapy once they have been diagnosed using normal medical methods. The original reasons for undertaking this study were simple. Many patients were asking about alternative therapies and it seemed only right to try to find out something about them. We also realised that very few of our colleagues knew much about the methods of these practitioners, although that has been changing gradually over the last five years.

It soon became clear that the whole area was a minefield. It is not difficult to find proponents of certain therapies who are quite uncritical about what they are doing, but that sometimes applies to all of us. For instance, we have seen people who have parted with a good deal of money for long courses of treatment which have done no good at all. Most alternative practitioners would say that if you have not noticed some effect after two or three sessions then it is probably not worth continuing. If you do get an effect, then the treatment may need to go on for very much longer. The other aspect of this uncritical approach was even more startling. We learned from one practitioner that 90 per cent of all depression was caused by food allergy, while another said that 90 per cent was caused not by food but by an alteration in the energy fields of the body. There were several other 90 per cents too! They cannot all be right. To many practitioners the underlying philosophy of their treatment is all important, but we have preferred to concentrate on results. A typically scientific and medical approach to be sure, but this is really what people are interested in, at least in the beginning.

Finally, a question is often asked — do we suggest or favour any particular form of therapy? The answer is most definitely no. We do not suggest alternative treatment but we try always to respond positively if the subject arises. It does seem clear that different forms of alternative medicine suit some people more than others, and if patients or their families are intent on trying these techniques, then we may try to point them in the right direction. We know that people will continue to go for alternative therapies whatever we and our colleagues may say about there being no proof that they work. We try to ensure that if patients do insist on having it, that it is done safely and well. We are all delighted if it does work — and work it often does.

CHAPTER FOUR

Acupuncture and Depression

In many respects acupuncture has become the flagship of the alternative medical therapies but it actually covers several separate practices. In the West, it is practised by three groups of people: doctors who have studied it, usually at post-graduate courses; physiotherapists and some nurses who also train after obtaining their initial qualification; and lay acupuncturists whose training varies enormously from those who have attended full-time courses lasting several years to those who have only taken correspondence courses.

The main type of acupuncture in use at the moment is traditional Chinese acupuncture, and it is this which you are most likely to encounter. There are a number of variants, including acupuncture analgesia, which is used for pain relief, and electro-acupuncture in which electrical stimuli are used with acupuncture needles. In the West, there has developed in recent years a form of acupuncture which just deals with symptoms instead of trying to deal with root causes. Although this can be very useful for treating muscular aches and pains, it is rarely of much use for treating depression. Since it is the most commonly available, we shall concentrate on the traditional Chinese form of acupuncture.

Chinese acupuncture has been in use for thousands of years. The first records are at least 2,000 years old but there is some evidence that it has existed for much longer. A long history is no proof that it works, but it does suggest that at least sometimes it does do some good. Totally ineffective treatments are seldom used for more than a short time. It is important to realise that acupuncture is only one element of Chinese medical treatment, and most traditional practitioners use not only acupuncture but also herbal treatments and massage at the same time. The whole system is based on a philosophy totally different from that of Western medicine. It relates illness to disturbances of energy in the body. In perfect health there is a harmony between the basic forces of Yin and Yang. This balance changes from day to day. The way that on some days we feel better and more energetic than on others is interpreted in this system to mean that the balance of energies in our bodies is varying from day to day. This poses a problem for the Western scientist. Nobody has ever managed to measure any sort of body energy. Do we assume, therefore, that it does not exist at all? Well, that would be the easy solution to this problem, but it would be far more sensible to reserve judgement and simply look at the treatment and its results.

Jane was an attractive, dark-haired 27-year-old who had been married to David, a travelling salesman, for three years. She worked in the typing pool of a large commercial company in North London. She had been fit and healthy until six months earlier when she started to lose weight, have headaches and experience episodes of diarrhoea in the mornings. She began to lose interest in life and finally her husband brought her to see her family doctor. Jane's doctor knew the family well. Her mother had been treated with antidepressants for many years, and Jane had herself had a brief depressive episode in her late teens soon after she started taking the oral contraceptive pill. That episode had stopped within weeks of stopping the pill. Since then she had had a number of minor episodes of depression but had been fine since meeting David. After establishing that there was nothing physically wrong with her, the doctor interviewed Jane and her husband at some length. Six months earlier, at the time when all this started, David's work had taken him to the north of England for several weeks and Jane started to convince herself that he would never return. Even when he did return, her normally outgoing personality did not. First she became profoundly disinterested in life. Then she started to neglect herself and the housework. As she described it herself many months later, it was almost as if she was trying to punish David for having ever gone away. Jane was quite seriously depressed and her doctor decided to treat her with an antidepressant. Within a month Jane was very much better but she still did not feel that she was back to her old self. She was also very worried that all this might happen again, and perhaps this too was holding up her recovery. A friend from work had been having severe headaches and had recently been much improved by acupuncture, and suggested that Jane should try this form of treatment. At first Jane was sceptical. Acupuncture might be fashionable, but the thought of those needles was rather off-putting. She was also concerned that her doctor would refuse to have anything more to do with her if she tried some other form of treatment. Finally, she did discuss it with her doctor, and to her surprise he supported the idea. She had a total of six treatments from the same acupuncturist who had treated her friend. He was a medical doctor who had done a three-month intensive course of training in China. For about two days after the first treatment she felt dreadful but then gradually improved. At the end of the course she felt better than she had in many years, and when she was seen some nine months later she appeared totally recovered. We cannot say what will happen to Jane in the long run, but she is convinced that acupuncture has changed the underlying depressive side of her nature. Perhaps this conviction will be strong enough to prevent any more episodes of depression in the future, or perhaps acupuncture has actually brought about some change in her, the nature of which, as yet, we do not fully understand.

The acupuncturist sees the body covered in several hundred carefully localised points which are joined together by lines or meridians. These are the energy channels of the body and it is claimed that it is possible to measure them electrically. We have met some practitioners who claimed to be able to see these channels running along the body, but none have yet demonstrated this to our satisfaction. Each one of these channels relates to a particular organ or system of the body. For instance, in depression it is quite common to work on the heart meridian. The story of the discovery of the acupuncture points and the meridians is largely shrouded in myth and mystery. There is no doubt, though, that many of the main acupuncture points become tender when disease effects some part of the body, and it may have been this which gave the first clue to their existence. It is the flow and the balance of the vital energy called Qi which now concerns the traditional practitioner. Depression is regarded as an imbalance of this energy, and the whole of the first part of the consultation is spent trying to establish the nature of the imbalance. It is thought that it weakens the body and makes it unable to resist the invasion of some outside agent. But while we might think in terms of a virus invading the body, the Chinese describe the invasion in terms of various types of weather. For example, a fever is described as a disease of heat, while the muscle aches of some viral infections are thought of as an invasion by wind. A totally different way of looking at disease, to be sure, but a little reflection shows that there is at least some similarity with the conventional view of illness.

Accurate diagnosis is the cornerstone of any form of treatment and in traditional Chinese medicine it requires great skill and experience. The visit to the acupuncturist invariably starts with a detailed history. At first this seems no different from the approach of the conventional doctor but soon it becomes clear that the whole slant of the questions is quite different. You will be asked about yourself in some detail. The effects of weather, the time at which your depression has been worse, the effects of food, and often a fair bit about your family. All the time the practitioner is listening not just to what you say but also to how you say it. Your expression, mood and speech are all regarded as being of crucial importance in helping to decide how you should be treated. Remember that the treatment which you finally receive will be tailor-made for you and so this lengthy personal approach is all important.

After this comes a physical examination which is totally different from any which you have had before. If you have an ache or pain somewhere, then that part may be looked at, but the key parts of the examination are based on the use of the pulse and the tongue for diagnosis. Pulse diagnosis is performed at the wrist. According to the ancient Chinese you have a total of twelve different pulses at the wrists. There are three deep and three superficial pulses on each side and each relates to a different organ or system of the body. Each of these is carefully examined, and classically each may vary in twelve different ways. As you can see, the possible variations are almost endless. Although this is the classical way of doing pulse diagnosis, it is extremely difficult to do well and requires many years of experience. Many practitioners have therefore been taught a modified form of pulse diagnosis which has been developed in China over the last few years. The pulse is still examined at the wrist, but instead of feeling at each of the twelve sites, the general character of the pulse is assessed. It is decided whether it is deficient or excessive in character, and this is taken to mean something about the state of the vital energy of the body. Recent evidence suggests that this newer method of using pulse diagnosis is almost as accurate as the older technique, especially when taken in conjunction with an accurate history and the final parts of the examination — tongue and smell. The use of smell is very common in all forms of diagnosis, which is not really surprising. It has been common knowledge for centuries that certain diseases are associated with particular bodily smells. The use of tongue diagnosis is particularly interesting. Although used to some extent in conventional medicine, the art of using the tongue to discover things about the working of the body reached its high point with the Chinese. The colour and character of the tongue is examined in some detail, together with its coating. So a tongue might be described as being red, furrowed, and weak, with a yellow coating. That may not sound too good, but most of us will have had a tongue like that at some time or other.

After this the acupuncturist is in a position to decide how he will treat you. Having made a diagnosis according to this system, he now uses a set of rules to decide exactly what he will do. These rules are based on the traditional concept of the functions of the organs, and the relationships of the organs to each other. For instance, the heart and its channel are involved in far more than just pumping blood around the body. They also have a major role in emotion and in the flow of the vital energy, Qi. There are a number of sophisticated systems which guide the acupuncturist in the selection of the correct points to treat. He may feel that the problem is one of an excess of heat or wind in the body, and there are particular points which are used to deal with this situation. Each of the different sets of rules relates to a fundamental part of ancient Chinese philosophy. The number five has great significance. According to old Chinese books, the rainbow is composed of five colours, and there are five elements, earth, fire, water, metal and wood. Each of the organ systems of the body represents one of these elements and there are special points on each of the meridians which can be used to stimulate or sedate the organ. There is a whole host of other rules which can be applied, but we have done enough to demonstrate the complexity of the system. Ultimately, the practitioner of acupuncture, like any other kind of therapist, relies largely on experience coupled with knowledge. But the treatment which you receive will invariably be different from that given to anyone else.

We come then to the treatment itself. We have all known people who are frightened or apprehensive about acupuncture purely because they think that it may hurt. Most of us have a few vague and unpleasant memories of painful injections in childhood. We must stress that acupuncture is, in skilled hands, virtually painless. (In the course of researching this book, the authors have tried most of the forms of therapy discussed, so we speak from personal experience!) The needles used in acupuncture are considerably smaller than those commonly used either for giving injections or for taking blood. They also have a rounded rather than a cutting point, so they rarely cause damage or bruising, and it is very uncommon to draw blood.

Usually the needles are applied to various points on the surface of the body. Many of the most commonly used points are located on the lower parts of the arms and legs. It has been claimed that this is because the Chinese do not like removing their clothes, and these are the only parts of the body which are accessible. Perhaps that is true, but according to the philosophy of acupuncture the actual reason has to do with the fact that some of the key points in the circulation of energy in the body are located in these areas. The other part of the body which is regarded as being of crucial importance is the ear. The use of the ear in acupuncture is a more recent innovation, although there is passing reference made to it in some very old Chinese manuscripts, and it has been said that it was used in ancient Egypt. Much of the development of ear acupuncture has taken place in Europe over the last thirty years, and is based on the idea that on the outside of the ear there is a kind of map of the human body. According to this map, most of the face and skull is represented on the ear-lobe, with the hand at the top, and the spine running around the large inner ridge of the ear. This all seemed rather far-fetched, but then in 1980 a scientific study was published which appears to give strong support to the idea. One of the authors of this book spent some time with a Chinese surgeon who routinely treated serious gall bladder pain by needling a particular point on the ear, and it did appear to be most effective. We have seen several patients with depression who have been treated almost exclusively with acupuncture to the ear, with some apparent success. Although one might imagine that having needles in the ear should be painful, in fact it does not seem to be.

It is believed that for maximum effect, it is necessary to obtain a needling sensation over each of the acupuncture points being used. This involves gently moving the needle while it is in the skin. The movement is very slight and it feels like a numb or dull sensation around the needle. Some people describe it as a feeling of warmth or even of bursting. It is rarely uncomfortable. It is interesting that sometimes the sensation moves up or down, and when it does this it follows one of the lines joining a group of acupuncture points. We have seen a patient who was needled in the foot, on one of the points on the liver channel, who almost immediately developed the needling sensation behind the eye, which is the other end of the channel. It is difficult to work out how this could happen if the channels did not exist, because there is no known nervous connection between the foot and the eye. So after the needles have been inserted they will be gently moved in this way and you will usually be asked what you feel. Sometimes the therapist will take your pulse again during the treatment and there may be some minor adjustments to the needles. They are usually left in for about 10 to 20 minutes, and the number used varies between four and twenty. Some of the pictures of treatment from China make it look as if the patient is a hedgehog with dozens of needles sticking out, but we have never seen this in the West.

Depending upon the treatment regime which has been decided

upon, the acupuncturist may also use moxibustion. This is a technique of applying local heat over an acupuncture point using the herb moxa. A compacted piece of the dried herb is stuck on the end of one of the acupuncture needles and lit. It smoulders and produces a cloud of aromatic smoke. This warms the needle and is supposed to provide a certain form of energy to the underlying acupuncture point and the associated channel. Although at one time people were deliberately burned and scarred with moxa, this is quite unnecessary and should never be done. We have not encountered any practitioners in the West who use such drastic measures.

By now you will be asking whether acupuncture is likely to help you. There are as yet no convincing scientific trials to show that it works in depression but, as we shall describe, there are undoubtedly people who have been greatly helped by it. If you ask the question at the beginning of the first treatment session, the practitioner will have to say that he cannot tell, at that stage, how you will respond. After the first treatment he should be developing a fairly good understanding of you as a person and be able to give you some idea of your chances of improvement. Although it is said that some people respond almost magically to only one treatment, we have never seen this in depression. If you do not feel any different after three treatments it is probably not worth continuing, but if you do, then it may be necessary to have a dozen treatments or more. Again everybody is different in their response and in the number of treatments they need. The next question is how often should you have treatment if it seems to be working? Again this varies, but the average is once a week. The Chinese normally go in for daily sessions, but this does not seem to have any particular advantage. People often show their greatest response to treatment in the hours and days afterwards, so the gap of a few days makes it easier to gauge the progress of the treatment.

Finally, can depression actually be cured with acupuncture? Well, as we have said, there is no good evidence one way or the other. The fact remains that we have seen several people who have maintained a remarkable improvement. What does seem clear is that many can be helped if not actually cured. Sometimes it is necessary to have a top up — another few treatments after a month or two, but that is not always the case. Quite often the traditional acupuncturist will give you some special herbs to continue taking from time to time. We really know very little about these herbs, but perhaps they do contain some form of active chemical compound. Some acupuncturists also use a form of massage based on the points and channels. We have seen one case where the therapist showed a patient's husband one or two simple massage techniques which she says helped her. We will, of course, never know whether it was the massage stimulating the energy of the body or the effect of the husband who finally gave his wife a good deal of time and attention.

Although we have seen quite a number of people who have responded very well to acupuncture treatment, we have also seen some failures.

Peter is a good example. A bearded 38-year-old schoolteacher from Yorkshire, Peter had settled in London after his marriage broke up five years earlier. A previously happy and contented man, he had never had any hint of any sort of problems and he was highly regarded as a teacher. Then it all changed. For ten years he had suffered from occasional episodes of depression, and this, combined with regular bouts of heavy drinking, came close to wrecking his career. He had few friends and distrusted the medical profession. He began to realise that he had to do something to help himself. He went to a practitioner who treated him for the best part of six months. At the end of this time there was no improvement. His sleep worsened and he felt increasingly hopeless. He was also some £400 poorer. Peter took a massive overdose of aspirin and very nearly died. He was subsequently treated by a conventional psychiatrist, is now back at work and is shortly going to remarry.

The case of Peter is important because it emphasises several of the points which we have raised. First, he was not being looked after by a doctor who should have been able to see that things were reaching breaking point. Second, he had a long course of treatment without apparent benefit, and continued because the practitioner kept assuring him that he was actually improving in some way. And, finally, the practitioner — he described himself as an acupuncturist but we were never able to establish what training he had had — was not listed on any of the professional registers. As we shall discuss with each of the alternative therapies, in many Western countries there are now registers of practitioners who have undergone a minimum training, and if you want to try one of these therapies, either ask your doctor if he will recommend someone or else find out whether a therapist is on the register. This is a good way both to find out if the person is adequately trained and to reassure yourself that he is likely to behave ethically. (We give some details of registers at the back of the book.)

Before we leave acupuncture, we should just consider one more thing. We have given a broad outline of how the acupuncturist thinks his treatment works. This explanation is impossible to understand in terms of conventional medical science. So if we assume that acupuncture does something more than just administer a hefty placebo, is there a possibility of some scientific explanation? Well, indeed there may be. It has been suggested that acupuncture works via hypnosis, but that suggestion does not really hold water. What is more likely is that in some way it alters the balance of various chemicals in the brain. In the final section of the book, we will be discussing the evidence that depression is related to changes in the balance of various chemicals in the brain. There is now good evidence that some types of acupuncture have effects on these same chemical systems. It is sobering to think that after 2,000 years we are probably about to prove that the Chinese were right all along, not just about the effectiveness of their methods but also about their diagnostic techniques. History-taking, the tongue and smell are all perfectly plausible to the Western scientist. A bigger problem is the idea of pulse diagnosis which we discussed earlier. There is nothing about the different pulses in standard medical textbooks. It is very interesting that within the last three or four years there has been some preliminary scientific evidence to suggest that these pulses actually exist. Pulse diagnosis is based upon centuries of careful observation, longer than the whole history of modern medicine. It would be staggering if there were nothing in it, but it seems amazing that only now might the West be catching up with this technique.

CHAPTER FIVE

Homoeopathy — A Good Alternative?

The use of homoeopathic medicine is growing very rapidly throughout the Western world. It is practised both by doctors and lay practitioners and homoeopathic remedies are freely available for use by the public. In Britain, homoeopathic treatment is available under the National Health Service, and there are now many doctors both in general practice and in the special homoeopathic hospitals who use it together with conventional treatments.

The basic ideas of homoeopathy have an ancient history, but the modern founder was Dr Samuel Hahnemann in the early part of the nineteenth century. Homoeopathic treatment is based on the use of the so-called 'similar principle', which has also been described as 'like cures like'. This involves the concept of treating an illness or disease with a remedy which may cause similar symptoms. We will explain this in a little detail because it is the key to understanding what happens when you go to see a homoeopathic practitioner. One of the early remedies discovered by Hahnemann illustrates the 'similar principle' rather well. He noticed that people who had malaria often had symptoms very similar to those of poisoning with cinchona bark — the old active ingredient of tonic water — so he decided to treat malaria patients with small amounts of cinchona. To everyone's surprise the patients recovered. What was still more surprising about his discovery was that the effect occurred even with very dilute solutions of cinchona. He demonstrated that even when the cinchona was diluted down until there was hardly any left in the remedy, he still observed effects. Since that time other homoeopaths have claimed that when the original substance is diluted several million times the effects of the remedy become stronger and not weaker.

The observation that poisoning with cinchona bark produces symptoms very similar to malaria formed the basis for the 'provings' of homoeopathy. Proving of remedies is something which is still going on today; healthy volunteers are given repeated small doses of a remedy and their reactions monitored. It is actually a perfectly safe procedure — the volunteers are not allowed to become overtly ill — but, nonetheless, patients are never used for this purpose. Homoeopaths have also examined the effects of poisoning with a large number of different agents. Much of this information had been in the medical literature for many years but Hahnemann and his followers extended it considerably. All this information has been put together into the homoeopathic Materia Medica, the grand list of all the remedies used. The key to this list is a large book called a 'repertory', which is an enormous list of symptoms.

The reason for putting all this effort into the examination of poisonings and the provings is the idea of like curing like. By studying information from these two sources it is possible to build up a picture of the symptoms characteristic of a remedy. When a patient consults a homoeopath the symptoms are compared with those of various remedies until a close match is found. This is the remedy which is used for treatment.

Carol was a 47-year-old shop assistant. In her teens she had done well at school and had planned to go to college. Then she had met a young butcher's apprentice and after a brief affair she had become pregnant. They married three months before her daughter was born but the marriage was a disaster and by the age of 23 she had divorced. She married again when she was 30 but again the marriage did not last. By the age of 35 she was divorced again and swore to have nothing more to do with men. The next twelve years were marked by repeated episodes of depression. Carol began to drink, and by the time that she was seen she was consuming two or three bottles of sherry a week and smoking twenty cigarettes each day. Her general practitioner had treated her with several courses of antidepressants and tranquillisers, but she refused psychiatric referral even when she seriously started to contemplate suicide. Her daughter had married some years earlier and lived a few miles away. It was finally her daughter who took her to see a homoeopathic doctor. He found Carol to be an intelligent but very depressed woman who admitted to having felt suicidal on many occasions. She had a marked lack of self-confidence and seemed restless and hurried. When asked about her failed marriages she was initially angry and uncommunicative, but she then revealed that she had always been irritable and would become furious if anyone contradicted her. She tended to be extremely critical and generally discontented with life. She was sleeping poorly and had recurrent nightmares in which she died or else fell from a great height. She had withdrawn from relationships, although several men had taken an interest in her over the last few years. The doctor found that she had very cold hands and feet, a dark brown tongue and catarrh. She admitted that despite the cold hands and feet she always felt better if she was in the open air. She was prescribed homoeopathic gold and was then seen for half an hour, once every three weeks for the next two months. Throughout this time she gradually improved. She stopped drinking except on social occasions, cut her cigarette consumption to four or five a day and felt more lively than she had done in many years. She has had no further episodes of depression and does not take any medications.

What happens when you go to see a homoeopath? The homoeopath goes into the details of the complaint rather more comprehensively than other practitioners might. He is also particularly concerned with other general symptoms which conventional medical practitioners may not link with depression in the same way. He will be interested to know, for example, how you react to cold or heat or extremes of these. Do you feel better in the open air or indoors? Do you you perspire a lot? Are there any times of the day when your depression seems particularly bad, and does weather have any effect on you? How do you sleep, and do you ever remember any particular dreams? Your tastes in food will also be relevant if you have strong likes or dislikes which are not influenced by advice, habit or religion.

These may be very helpful in deciding on the remedy for you. From all this he will build up a total picture of you, constructed of two closely linked parts. One part is your constitutional type — this is similar to what psychologists refer to as your personality 'traits', those life-long emotional predispositions to things. The other part is your current situation, which is largely dependent on your depression. It is this which varies all the time during your life and will continue to change as treatment proceeds. It roughly corresponds to what psychologists call your personality 'state'.

The homoeopath is particularly interested in the onset of the illness, even if this was many years earlier. Did the depression first start after the loss of a loved one, or after some profound emotional experience or anger? It may even have started after a fall or after a fright — things which the conventional doctor would think of minor importance. Perhaps there may be something to suggest a long-standing smouldering resentment which is underlying the depression. These questions are not just asked because of their psychological implications but also because they may point towards specific remedies. There will also be questions about family history, especially whether there are any diseases which run in the family. There is no need to worry if you cannot answer all the questions, all medical practitioners know how difficult it is to remember everything in detail. After all this extensive history-taking, the homoeopathic physician can proceed to the next stage. He will usually consult the repertory. This contains many thousands of symptoms, and by cross-checking your symptoms against those in the book he arrives at the right remedy. It is remarkable that this process, which takes a few minutes, will almost invariably point to just one remedy from the 2,000 or so which are listed. Some homoeopaths now use a small computer to help them find the correct remedy, and more will probably do so in the future. There are occasions when the history is so clear cut that it is not necessary to go the repertory.

All that is now left is to decide on the correct dose. Often you will only be given a single dose of the remedy and then left alone for three or four weeks to see what happens. Many of the potent remedies are best given in this way because, unlike conventional treatments, taking more of a remedy does not add to the benefit which it may have for you. There are several possible results of homoeopathic treatment: you may have no effect at all; you may transiently become worse; or you may improve. The homoeopath also looks for variations on these themes and they will determine what is done next. There is little relationship between the severity of the symptoms and your response.

At your second consultation, the homoeopath will again take a brief history in order to establish whether you have had a reaction. He will then decide if you should have a further dose, or some different remedy, or perhaps he will leave you a while longer without interfering.

The history in Carol's case fitted very well with the result of the provings of metallic gold and so this was the only remedy which would really have been of use. It is this selection of a treatment on the basis of a matching of the patient's symptoms with the symptom picture of the remedy which lies at the heart of homoeopathic practice.

Although the remedy that is used will be tailor made to your requirements, there are a small number of homoeopathic remedies that are used more often than others in the treatment of depression. In mild cases of depression they can be bought over the counter and used, without the need for going to a homoeopath. They are harmless in themselves, and if you take the wrong remedy it will just not work. Side-effects probably never happen except perhaps with the very potent preparations, which you will not be sold unless on prescription. Although the remedies themselves are safe, we must again make the point that one potential problem about using the remedies is that you may continue to take them when in fact you need some other form of treatment. It is the usual practice to take only one remedy at a time, but some practitioners may use remedies in combination. It is not clear whether the single remedy idea is important or not, and different homoeopaths have different views on this.

For historical reasons the remedies are typically given Latin names, and we now give details of a few of them.

We have already mentioned the use of homoeopathic gold, which is called *Aurum metallicum* when it is dispensed. Carol showed many of the typical features of *Aurum*. She had suicidal depression with a lack of confidence, and she became angry and irritable if contradicted. She was discontented and preferred the open air, despite having cold hands and feet. These are all symptoms straight out of the homoeopathic Materia Medica for gold. The remedy was arrived at by simply taking a list of Carol's symptoms and then going through the repertory. For each symptom there are several separate remedies listed. By noting the remedies attached to each symptom, the homoeopath quickly finds that one particular remedy is common to each symptom. It is this which is ultimately used. Each remedy has an enormous number of symptoms attached to it. All these symptoms are based on many years of observation, so not surprisingly some of the collections of symptoms would also be recognised by practitioners of the younger science of conventional medicine. Taking our example of homoeopathic gold, the standard reference work lists over five pages of symptoms. These include all Carol's symptoms, and also bad breath, chest pain, skin rashes, disorders of smell and pains in the bones. Not all of these will be present in the person who is treated with gold, but many will, and it is by a careful assessment of the important symptoms that the homoeopath finally decides what to use for treatment. It is also important to note that the same remedy may occasionally be used for treating people who do not have depression at all. They may, for instance, have the combination of bad breath, rashes and chest pain, and the repertory might lean towards gold as the remedy. For the homoeopath the actual complaint is not as important as all the other things which you tell him, and how you tell it.

Another commonly used remedy, especially for women with depression, is *Cimicifuga*. People who need this remedy usually have a profound fear of death and their depression is characterised by an awful gloom. They feel that there is a great black cloud hovering over them and find it difficult to sleep. They are often talkative, restless, irritable and suspicious, with pale faces and dark rings under the eyes, and they flush very easily. There is marked sensitivity to cold and damp.

Patients who need *Phosphoric acid* tend to be remarkably indifferent to everything. Not only are they depressed but they are listless and apathetic. They do not seem to want anything and do not even want to talk. They cannot collect their thoughts properly and often have odd aches and pains in various parts of the body. It is sometimes possible to trace back the trouble to some event like homesickness or a disappointing relationship.

Natrum Sulphuricum is often used in depression if there is a past history of a head injury, or if the person has asthma or pneumonia. These people tend to be very tearful, and music may make them feel sad or even weep. They are perhaps tired of life but do not actually want to end it. Typically they are irritable first thing in the morning and hate having to speak or be spoken to for the first hour or two after getting out of bed.

Drosera is a remedy that is often given to children with whooping cough, but it is often used in the treatment of depression in adults, particularly if there is a past history of tuberculosis. There is often a marked feeling of dejection about what they feel others have done to them in the past. They tend to feel generally disheartened about the future, and have ideas that they are being deceived by spiteful, envious people. Some of them can become quite enraged over very minor things, they are restless and find it difficult to stick at anything for any length of time.

Psorinum is a remedy which is usually used for treating skin disease but is also often used in treating depression. People who might benefit from this remedy are those who feel generally hopeless and are full of all sorts of fears and forebodings. These often tend to focus on work or business and there is a great fear that the business will fail. They may even have nightmares about work and tend to feel physically cold all the time.

A final remedy which is often used in treating depression is *Calcarea Carbonica*. We have seen a case where this was used most effectively.

Gerald was a 37-year-old accountant. The most noticeable thing on meeting him was that he was a rather pale and flabby individual, his hands were soft and damp and his neck looked rather scraggy. Everything about him was slow. He moved slowly, and both his speech and his intellect seemed lethargic. It was difficult to imagine how he managed to do his job, and over the last few months his work performance had gone steadily downhill. He had become progressively more depressed and had started worrying about the smallest things. He lived in perpetual fear that something dreadful was going to happen. He had always been a bit like this but it had become worse quite suddenly after a bad attack of influenza the previous winter. He consulted his general practitioner, who regularly used homoeopathic treatments as well as conventional medications. He felt that there was a possibility that Gerald had an underactive thyroid gland, and he first proved that this was not the case. There are a small number of specific remedies which are used after viral infections, but on this occasion the doctor decided that Gerald was such a good example of a *Calcarea Carbonica* type that he decided to use this to treat him. The effect was quite remarkable. Within two weeks of starting treatment he said that he felt a new man. He started to speed up mentally and physically and his depression lifted completely. He has subsequently remained fit and healthy.

The authors had a considerable difficulty in deciding whether to include any details of remedies in this book. We have seen them work, but that is very different from suggesting that you should try them blindly without supervision. We might perhaps agree once we have seen and assessed a patient ourselves, but the problem is always that it takes an expert in depression to know when the situation is getting out of hand. Common sense is normally enough to say when depression is mild or severe, or when it is just a mood disorder, but common sense is not always a reliable guide. We stick to the idea that if depression needs *any* form of treatment, then it should first be assessed by someone who is used to dealing with the problem. We know that there are some people who will take these remedies anyway and for them we present some simple guidelines. If you are going to try to use homoeopathic remedies, you should look for either the 12C or 30C potencies. When you take the remedy, you place it in your mouth and let it slowly dissolve. It is said that you should not smoke or use strong toothpaste for the hour or so before you take the remedy.

In Britain, if you want to have homoeopathic treatment, your general practitioner can refer you, and you can have free treatment under the National Health Service. Alternatively he or she may suggest a non-medical homoeopath and the usual rule applies about finding somebody who is trained and registered. (We give details about this at the end of the book.)

The idea of like treating like is still regarded with considerable scepticism by the medical profession in general, but the principle is actually used in parts of conventional medicine, notably in vaccination and some cancer therapy. What is more difficult to understand is the apparent therapeutic effect of the infinitesimally small doses which are used in homoeopathy. The basic substance from which the remedy is made may be of animal, vegetable or mineral origin. The raw material is crushed and an alcoholic extract made by a process of soaking and filtering. Then begins the process of making the diluted homoeopathic remedy. One drop of the alcoholic extract is added to ten or a hundred drops of alcohol or an alcohol and water mixture. It is then vigorously shaken either by hand or by machine. It is this shaking which is regarded as the important part of making a homoeopathic remedy — the preparation is more than just making dilutions. Some remedies which are insoluble are made instead using lactose powder as the diluting substance. The diluting process is continued for a standard number of times to produce the final remedy which can be prescribed. There are certain standard dilutions which are used in practice. Most often these are the so-called 6C, 12C or 30C preparations which can be bought over the counter in many pharmacies, and even in some health food shops. The C means that the remedy has been diluted a hundredfold at each stage in its preparation. The number indicates how many times this dilution has been carried out. With the 12C preparation, the dilution of one drop in a hundred drops has been carried out twelve times, so the final product has been diluted to such an extent that one part of the original now exists in 1,000,000,000,000 parts of the solution. The 12C and 30C preparations do not actually contain any of the original substance, and the problem for the medical scientist is the idea that something which contains just alcohol and water can have any kind of effect on the mind. Other even more dilute remedies designated 1M and 10M are often prescribed and it is said that these are even more potent. It does seem that this principle of increasing potency with increasing dilution is contrary to common sense. But many ideas that have at first seemed illogical have ultimately been shown to have some sense in them. Rather than worrying about the logic of the idea, it is more sensible to have a look at the evidence. At the moment there is not much apart from simple uncontrolled observations, but it will be important for all of us to keep an open mind in the future if we are to avoid losing potentially valuable treatments.

Anecdotes about the effectiveness of homoeopathy do not cut much ice with the sceptic. So, is there any evidence that homoeopathic treatment actually works? There have been many attempts to show that the potentised remedies have effects in the laboratory, and some of them seem now to demonstrate that there is an effect which cannot be explained using our normal scientific model. All of these experiments are being repeated at the moment and so we must wait to see if scientists can repeat these experiments. Others have been performing a number of clinical trials on homoeopathic remedies, and it does look as if some remedies do have a significant effect which cannot be explained away on the basis of a placebo response. There have not yet been any trials of homoeopathy in depression and so we cannot give a scientific answer to the question, does it work? All we can say is that our observations lead us to think that homoeopathy may be a valuable treatment in some people.

CHAPTER SIX

Depression, Food, Nutrition and Vitamins

Acupuncture and homoeopathy represent two complete treatment systems. We turn now to a group of alternative medical treatments that between them may perhaps turn out to be the most important of all therapeutic innovations. We are referring to abnormal reactions to food and the role of faulty nutrition as a cause of depression. Normally these two are dealt with separately but there are so many points of contact between them that we have decided to discuss them together.

The idea that food sensitivity may be a causative factor in disease is by no means new, and some alternative practitioners have been applying the concept for a very long time. Practitioners who deal with these problems are referred to as clinical ecologists. It is only recently that this approach towards the causes and treatment of disease has started to draw the attention of the medical profession.

First, let us be quite clear about what we mean by food sensitivity. We have all heard a great deal in the popular press about 'food allergy'. It is suggested that some people are allergic to food in the same way that hay fever sufferers, who get a runny nose when the pollen count is high, are allergic to pollen. In the vast majority of patients who are sensitive to food, there is no evidence of an actual allergy of the type that one gets in hay fever. They do not have any of the chemical changes in their bodies which accompany an allergic reaction. This is an important point when trying to treat food-sensitive patients.

There are several different types of food sensitivity. One of the best known is the triggering of migraine by foods like cheese and chocolate in some predisposed people. The aspect of food sensitivity which most concerns us here is the development of emotional changes associated with particular foods. We must stress that this does not mean the sort of reaction that you get if you are forced to eat something which you hate, which comes under the heading of food aversion. It means the generalised psychological and perhaps physical response which follows the exposure to certain foods and chemicals.

So why should anybody be sensitive to food? Despite a lifetime of eating, most of us never have any noticeable problem. The intestines have developed a remarkable system for defending us against most types of food, but in some people there are foods which can slip through the net — not the foods themselves, but certain chemical constituents which they contain. These may be either a part of the food itself or some additive that is put in during preparation. Many people find that they become sensitive to certain foods at various times, notably when they are run down. Some women only become food sensitive just before their menstrual period. So both the chemical constituents of foods and the make-up of the person eating them contribute to food sensitivity.

To get an idea of what happens in food sensitivity, it is useful to consider how the body reacts if it is exposed to irritant substances — we shall take alcohol as an example. If you are not used to drink, when you first take some alcohol it causes several symptoms; it is a poison, and causes an upset stomach, flushing and headache. A little may relax you and make you feel good but an excess makes you drunk. It is also an important cause of depression. If you avoid further alcohol, all the symptoms settle quite rapidly, but if you continue to drink the body initially adapts to the alcohol, until you reach the stage where the body can no longer adapt and then you develop chronic symptoms. This is probably what happens with food sensitivity as well. Everything is fine unless your make-up makes you susceptible, and then your body can no longer adapt. If you then stop taking in the food or alcohol, your body may react with a whole new set of symptoms — there may actually be withdrawal symptoms. Many clinical ecologists consider that if you have a craving for a particular food, then you may actually be sensitive to it. This becomes very important when trying to establish whether someone is sensitive to a particular food.

There is a lot of discussion about how common food sensitivity may be. We said earlier that we had met people who claimed that 90 per cent of all depression stemmed from this problem, but most practitioners with experience in this area feel that the figure is a good deal lower. From a review of the practitioners that we have met, and of the books and scientific papers on the subject, we estimate that food or chemical sensitivity makes a major contribution to less than 10 per cent of all cases of depression, but may be a factor in many more. We readily acknowledge that any such figures remain speculative until formal research is done.

The chance then of some food sensitivity being the cause of your depression is not actually very high. Any examination of a possible food element in depression must be done very carefully. There is no point at all in going on endless special diets in the hope of curing depression Although there are some practitioners who do this sort of thing, it is a practice which is in no one's best interests. Our usual rule applies, either have a look at this problem yourself, under medical supervision, or seek the advice of a reputable practitioner, and do not go on with the approach unless you rapidly see a positive benefit. It is also important to emphasise that any form of special diet must be nutritionally sound — you must still get the correct amounts of vitamins and minerals. If in doubt discuss it with your doctor.

So how does a clinical ecologist set about making a diagnosis of food sensitivity?

The most commonly used technique is the elimination diet. This starts with a five-day period when the patient is put on a fast, during which he is only allowed to take spring water. Some practitioners are rather less strict and allow a diet of lamb and pears during this period. These two foods rarely cause food sensitivity, perhaps because lamb is less adulterated by chemical treatments than most other meats, and pears are not treated with so many chemicals while they are growing. It is assumed that this fast both cleans out the body, to rid it of harmful foods already eaten, and makes you particularly susceptible to any foods which may be causing trouble. Foods are then reintroduced one at a time, with each meal consisting of one food only. It is generally recommended that rarely eaten foods should be reintroduced first. These are unlikely to be the cause of the problem, and this method thus allows a more varied diet to be arrived at fairly quickly. The patient is allowed to continue eating each food which has not caused any immediate symptoms. Although people vary quite a lot, there are certain foods which are said to be incriminated in depression more often than others. These in approximate order of frequency are:

Alcohol
Wheat
Milk and dairy produce
Coffee
Corn or maize
Citrus fruits

It is said that the frequency of finding different foods which cause depression is related to the amount of the food which is eaten in the population and this may give some clues as to the mechanism of food sensitivity. This may explain why the lists of foods are different in some American books, since there are substantial differences in some elements of European and American diets. According to clinical ecologists, people who are food sensitive are usually sensitive to more than one food at a time.

Many different techniques are used for assessing whether someone is sensitive to the food which he has just eaten. The obvious one is to see if symptoms of depression occur after a meal, but this is unreliable since such symptoms may take quite some time to develop. Because of the time lag in the development of symptoms, the whole approach of using exclusion diets always seems rather a hit or miss way of tackling the problem, but it remains the easiest one for the individual to try. Another approach which has many supporters is to take the pulse immediately after eating a specified food. This again is usually done after a fast. It is said that the pulse speeds up if you have just been exposed to a food which causes trouble. This is rather unreliable and non-specific and we have yet to be convinced that it has much value.

As with homoeopathic remedies, we feel that this may be a most valuable approach but it must be carefully monitored, and done only after consultation with a competent physician. If you feel that you want to investigate the possibility that foods may be implicated, then clinical ecologists would say that it is best to go in for the five-day fast and to follow up by reintroducing one food a day. They would usually suggest starting at the top of the list and working your way down. Naturally, if there are some foods which you never touch anyway, then it would not be necessary to experiment with those.

Many clinical ecologists allege that there are a whole host of chemicals in the environment which may cause depression in susceptible individuals. These include petrol fumes, perfumes, pesticides, and the fumes given off by gas cookers. We have not so far seen any patients who were definitely sensitive to any of these agents, although there are many clinical ecologists who claim that they are a common cause of depression. If you do happen to notice that you become depressed after exposure to one of these agents, it would be necessary for this to be formally tested by a medical specialist, rather than to try experimenting on your own.

If you should decide to pursue this approach by going to see a clinical ecologist, there are several other tests which may be used to see if you are food or chemical sensitive. All of these are said to have helped patients, but all of them are awaiting scientific validation.

A commonly used test is the so-called RAST test, which stands for radio-allergosorbent test — a long name for a test which is designed to prove whether or not you have antibodies in your blood. Antibodies normally exist to protect you against harmful agents in the environment, most commonly bacteria. They have a number of other actions, but the idea is that in food sensitivity you may develop antibodies against food. It is in common use, but not only is it a difficult test to do well, but the findings may not be all that relevant to you. Some people have positive tests to foods which have never given them a day's trouble.

Over the last few years a number of other techniques have been used to investigate food sensitivity. They are all unorthodox in the extreme and we have yet to be convinced that any of them are of much use. They include tests in which an extract of the food is squirted under the tongue or injected into the skin, and various types of electrical testing.

Despite the problems of doing and interpreting the RAST and other tests, the evidence is beginning to suggest that we may soon be able to identify and treat patients who are genuinely food sensitive. It is important to do this because many who think that they are food sensitive are definitely not.

It is possible that food sensitivities may cause chemical changes in the body, a closely related problem is hypoglycaemia or low blood sugar. Normally your blood sugar is carefully maintained at a certain level which is needed for the normal functioning of your body. In recent years, there has been much debate about whether it is possible for people to get physical and mental symptoms if their blood sugar drops during the hours after a meal. We have known for years that patients who are being treated with insulin or tablets for diabetes may drop their blood sugar and develop a whole group of symptoms, from sweating and palpitations to unconsciousness. Most physicians still consider that it cannot happen in people unless they are taking these drugs, because the body has extremely efficient mechanisms for maintaining a stable blood glucose level. Despite this, we have now seen a small number of depressed patients whose symptoms have gone completely when they have adjusted their diet in order to maintain a stable blood sugar level throughout the day.

Eleanor was an intelligent 21-year-old art student. She had never had any health problems but had recently been experiencing a number of episodes of mild depression and lethargy for no very obvious reason. She admitted that she felt tired most of the time and had recently found it more and more difficult to finish some of her work. Eleanor lived in a flat in East London with some fellow students, was happy with her steady boyfriend and apart from minor financial worries her life was going well. She had a physical examination by the college doctor and nothing could be found. Routine blood tests, including a blood sugar check, were all normal. On close questioning, it appeared that Eleanor had for some time noticed feelings of intense tiredness in the mornings before lunch, and again in the early evenings. Her hands sometimes shook so badly that she could not do her work and she would feel nauseated. She smoked four or five cigarettes each day and drank a moderate amount of alcohol. She ate poorly and infrequently, normally taking a cup of coffee before she left for college in the mornings. She then had nothing further until lunchtime when she would eat some sandwiches. The time and content of the evening meal varied enormously but was usually high in carbohydrate and fat. It was thought possible that she might be experiencing episodes of low blood sugar and her diet was totally reorganised. She was instructed to eat little and often and to avoid coffee, refined (white) bread and sugar. She was also asked to cut down on her alcohol consumption. Within one week Eleanor was back to normal and she has had no further episodes of lethargy or depression.

It would be easy to say that Eleanor's symptoms hnd nothing to do with the dietary manipulations, and that there was some other factor. In any case, although she was diagnosed as having depression, many psychiatrists would just say that she had episodes of depressed mood rather than full-blown depression. But her case is by no means unique. Some practitioners, particularly in the United States, use a chemical test to help them diagnose this condition, in which you take a measured quantity of glucose on an empty stomach, and then have blood tests done hourly for five hours. The idea behind the test is that if people have a large quantity of glucose, the level of the sugar in the blood rises normally. But in hypoglycaemics, in the hours after this it falls dramatically. It is this fall in blood sugar which is said to cause the symptoms of hypoglycaemia. There remains some doubt about the usefulness of this test, and it is not yet recommended except in a very small number of depressives who clearly have physical symptoms of low blood sugar.

Taking large amounts of alcohol or rapidly absorbed sugars in the diet means that the blood sugar level bounces up and down throughout the day, and may cause symptoms. Nobody knows how common this problem may be amongst patients with depression, and it is being researched at the moment.

As far as individual people are concerned, it is sometimes difficult to make the diagnosis. Self-diagnosis is very difficult and, we feel, potentially dangerous. But what can be done is to eat sensibly. What we recommend is that you should follow the general advice given to Eleanor:

1 If you drink alcohol, cut down your consumption.
2 Eat little and often.
3 Avoid white sugar, white bread and white rice.
4 Cut down your consumption of sweet and fatty foods.
5 Eat more high fibre and fresh fruits and vegetables.

This represents an outline of the sort of healthy diet which you should be on, even if you have not got hypoglycaemia.

We come now to another form of alternative medical treatment for depression, one which is being actively explored by a number of members of the medical profession and some distinguished scientists. This is the concept that depression, and indeed a number of medical disorders, may be caused by an imbalance in certain metals in the body, or else by a vitamin deficiency. Although most doctors still regard these theories as quite groundless, there is some evidence that depression can sometimes be eradicated by correcting these imbalances.

Several different vitamin deficiencies have been said to occur in depression, but here we come up against the problem for the medical scientist. We have known for over a hundred years that there are certain illnesses that can be caused by vitamin deficiency, and we can measure most vitamin levels in the blood. The routine measurements of vitamins are usually normal in depression, so how can people say that you might be deficient in a certain vitamin? Well, the idea is that although you might have perfectly normal levels of the vitamin in your blood, the rest of your body may not have enough. The idea has developed that what you may need is a big dose of particular vitamins, both to restock your body, and also to correct imbalances between the different vitamins, which may be just as bad as being deficient in one. Sceptics say that there is no point in taking vitamins for non-existent deficiencies, and most of the vitamins are not even absorbed. This argument has been going on for twenty years, so let us just look at the theories in more detail.

In the past there was one type of vitamin deficiency which had enormous consequences. For hundreds of years the navies of the world suffered the ravages of scurvy, which sometimes incapacitated half the crew. In the 1740s it was discovered that scurvy could be avoided by eating limes. Some fifty years later it was adopted as policy in the British Navy and scurvy was wiped out at sea. Still later is was discovered that it was the vitamin C in limes which prevented scurvy. Now, every medical student knows the symptoms of scurvy, and most people with depression do not have them. Despite this, treatment with large doses of vitamin C (3,000 milligrams per day) has been said to be very beneficial in some patients. Is it just our old friend the placebo response or is there something more to it? For the final answer we will have to await the results of proper clinical trials, but you can do something useful for yourself in the interim. Although at several points in this chapter we will recommend that you keep an adequate vitamin intake, we must stress that you should not exceed the stated doses. In recent years there have been several reports of people who did themselves harm by taking enormous quantities of vitamins and such practices must be avoided.

Some practitioners have stated that depression may be caused by a mild deficiency of the vitamin B1, or thiamine. This sort of depression is associated with irritability, emotional instability, apathy, poor appetite and tingling in the fingers and toes. All these symptoms may have many different causes, but in some people who have this group of symptoms together they do improve markedly if they are treated with thiamine. It is very interesting that some doctors claim that drinking a lot of coffee causes you to lose thiamine, and that may be one reason why drinking excess coffee causes depression in some people. It also leads us to an important point. You may develop a chronic vitamin imbalance despite being on an apparently normal Western diet. Some foods may prevent the absorption of key vitamins, while others, like coffee, cause you to lose a vitamin in the urine. Doctors who use high-dose vitamin therapy recommend that people with depression should take 500 milligrams twice a day for one week, and thereafter should stay on 50 milligrams each day. This dose will not do any harm, and may perhaps do some good. If you do decide to go in for the vitamin approach, it is probably best to take a combination of all the vitamins which we shall be mentioning here, and if you have had no effect in one month then there is probably no point in continuing.

Gross deficiency of the vitamin niacin (nicotinic acid) leads to the clinical condition known as pellagra, one that is distressingly common amongst the starving and sometimes in the elderly, but is rarely seen in the affluent West. Nonetheless, there are some who say that mild niacin deficiency does occur in many despite having an apparently normal diet. One of the cardinal symptoms of mild niacin deficiency is depression. The average daily requirement of niacin is around 20 milligrams for men and 15 milligrams for women. You can normally get ample in our diet by eating fish or poultry or brewer's yeast. If it is being used in depression it is normally used in a dose of 50 milligrams twice a day, although some people use very much higher doses than this. There are a few situations in which high doses of niacin may be harmful, namely in diabetes, where it may elevate blood sugar, and in people being treated for high blood pressure in whom blood pressure may fall suddenly. If in doubt, check with your doctor.

There is one vitamin which some practitioners use quite often in the treatment of depression. This is pyridoxine or vitamin B6. You usually need only 3 milligrams of this vitamin each day, but when it is used for treatment, far larger doses are administered. The depression of pyridoxine deficiency is associated with explosive and sometimes quite hysterical episodes, though these people often tend to be rather shy. In women, premenstrual depression often responds well to treatment with pyridoxine with a dose of 150 milligrams per day. (In the final chapter of this book we shall be discussing why it might be of value in some people.)

The vitamin pantothenic acid is known to be of crucial importance in the body. It is a component of a particular chemical known as co-enzyme A. Classic textbooks deny the existence of any deficiency syndrome involving pantothenic acid, but some doctors have used it successfully to treat people with depression. We normally obtain pantothenic acid from a whole variety of foods, but excessive processing may lead to the destruction of much of the pantothenic acid content. Treatment with this vitamin usually needs 250 milligrams twice a day, again far in excess of the amount normally required.

Several other vitamins have been implicated in depression, but the only other one which we have seen used is vitamin A. This is found in large amounts in cod liver oil, which is a cheap and easy way to take the vitamin. Deficiency of vitamin A is supposed to cause tiredness and difficulties in sleeping in addition to depression. Many have recently become interested in the fact that this vitamin will lower the cholesterol level in the blood if taken for a prolonged period. It is usually used in the dose of 25,000 IU each day. A word of caution here: it is possible to get vitamin A toxicity if you take too much, and this is the maximum dose which you should take for any period of time, unless it is specifically recommended by a doctor. Children are often given vitamin A routinely in cod liver oil and they are usually not allowed more than 3,000 IU each day.

Some vitamins have an intimate relationship with certain metals in the body. Some of these exist in the body in vanishingly small amounts, and are known as trace metals. There are several of these, but the two which have been most often implicated in depression are copper and zinc. There appears to be a loose connection between these two; as the zinc level in the body rises, the copper level falls and vice versa. It is claimed that a high copper level may cause depression, and lowering the level improves it. So, if this is true, then where does copper come from? It is common in the environment, and its level is watched, at least in some countries. You may take in more in industrial pollution, in cigarettes, and from copper pipes.

It is difficult with conventional techniques to establish a trace metal deficiency or excess. A new and controversial technique is to take a specimen of hair and measure the levels of toxic and trace metals present in it. This is supposed to give an accurate idea of your bodily state because the metals are incorporated into the hair as it grows. The technique is not yet widely available. If it can be shown to be a valid way of showing something useful, then we may hear a great deal more about it in the future. In the absence of any easy way of discovering whether or not you have a problem with your metal status, we have heard two pieces of advice from the experts in this field:

1 Do not smoke, apart from everything else it draws some toxic metals into your lungs.
2 If you have copper pipes in the house, then run the tap for a few moments in the morning before drinking any water.

If we were running a court of law, we would have to say that nobody can yet prove the case that vitamins and minerals may be a cause of depression. Despite this it is true that we have seen patients who have benefited enormously from this approach to their treatment. It also seems that this sort of approach is particularly useful for those with very mild depression, who would like to try something for themselves. While all the benefit that we have seen may just be another example of a placebo reaction, it is alleged by practitioners specialising in this area that there is a quick and safe way for you to investigate this yourself.

As usual, if you are on treatment, continue with it and discuss your plan with your doctor. Ensure that you are taking a sensible diet. We have already given you some pointers on this. Then, the experts would suggest, for one month take the following high-dose vitamin schedule:

Vitamin A 25,000 IU per day.
Vitamin C 3,000 milligrams per day.
Pyridoxine (vitamin B6) 150 milligrams per day.
Niacin (nicotinic acid) 150 milligrams per day.
Pantothenic acid 250 milligrams twice a day.
Thiamine (vitamin B1) 500 milligrams twice a day for one week followed by 50 milligrams each day.

Most of these are available in combination tablets, and can be readily obtained from most pharmacists and health food stores. If you do have a useful effect from this regime, it is said that it should be possible for you to stop the vitamins after the month is up, and allow your diet to take over.

This way of using high-dose vitamins is very much a cookbook approach. Many of those who are firm believers in this way of treating depression use a far more tailor-made approach, which may well be better. None of us can judge until the research data have been presented. If your doctor decides that this is a reasonable approach for you to adopt, then remember that there are dangers in taking in too many vitamins, so do not exceed the amounts stated here.

CHAPTER SEVEN

Hypnosis

For a long time hypnosis was regarded with suspicion and hostility. In recent years, it has come to be seen as a relatively respectable form of treatment for a wide range of illnesses, emotional and psychological conditions, and personality problems. In the West, it is primarily practised by doctors or dentists who have had special training, or by clinical psychologists who are usually attached to hospital psychiatric departments. There are also a number of lay hypnotherapists in practice but the quality and quantity of their training is very variable.

Hypnosis has been used in some form or other throughout history. It has a fascinating past but a discussion of it lies outside the scope of this book. (The interested reader may pursue the references at the back.) There is a wealth of scientific data to prove its effectiveness. Many ask whether it is of use in the treatment of depression. The answer is that it is sometimes very useful indeed, although it should never be used alone as a treatment for depression. It has to be used in combination with some other approach, either a drug treatment or psychotherapy. Throughout this section on alternative approaches to treatment, we have emphasised that treatments could be done by lay practitioners so long as there was medical supervision. With hypnosis, we feel that it should only be done by competent, qualified practitioners and then only as one part of a treatment. It is a powerful technique, and this is no place for the amateur. Hypnosis is particularly valuable for helping the anxiety which sometimes accompanies depression, or in analysing some of the root causes of depression.

Until recently, hypnosis had a very poor press. There were

highly inaccurate representations of it in films and the media, and many still associate it with something vaguely sinister. It must be emphasised that therapeutic hypnosis cannot be administered against your will. You actually remain in control of yourself throughout the hypnotic session. It is a method of enabling you to use the powers of your own mind but there is nothing mystical about it. It is a technique that can be successfully learnt by most people, and the hypnotist does not require any special personality traits. Similarly, although some people are better hypnotic subjects than others, it is rare to find someone who genuinely cannot by hypnotised. There is absolutely no connection between the ease with which someone can be hypnotised and either their intelligence or gullibility.

In many respects, the hypnotic state is rather like the earliest stage of sleep. Some of the normal critical faculties of the mind are partially suspended, and it becomes possible for the hypnotherapist to communicate with your subconscious mind, without the interference of the intellect. We normally all have a number of barriers which may prevent contact with the deeper parts of ourselves. It is these barriers which we can sometimes get round by using hypnosis. It must be stressed that hypnosis is only an appropriate form of treatment in a minority of people with depression.

Daphne was an untidy, chain-smoking, greying woman in her early 40s who had a very long history of depression going back to her late teens. She had had several courses of treatment with antidepressant drugs, and had recently been referred to a psychiatrist as an out-patient. For a long time she had refused psychiatric help, although she did not seem to object to taking medications prescribed by her general practitioner. In the last few months she had been made redundant from her factory job. Then her common-law husband had left her after many years of a turbulent relationship. She had always slept poorly, but recently she had been sleeping very little and having nightmares from which she awoke screaming. She was sweaty and had lost weight. With these new symptoms it had been wondered if she might have an overactive thyroid gland but tests had shown that this was not the cause of her symptoms. The psychiatrist that she saw was an experienced hypnotherapist. He began Daphne's treatment in the conventional way with antidepressant medications and psychotherapy. He felt that there would be some value in using hypnosis, both to help with her symptoms of anxiety and to help him to discover something more about the deeper problems in her mind. She was an excellent hypnotic subject and her anxiety symptoms responded well. She was then gradually encouraged to become involved in helping herself with analysis, with quite good results. She was still undergoing treatment when last seen.

If it is decided to treat you with hypnosis, it will probably take place in the normal consulting room. You will first be made comfortable, usually sitting in a chair. Sometimes you will be asked to lie on a couch, just because this can be still more comfortable. It is helpful if the room is kept at a comfortable temperature and the lighting dimmed.

Hypnotherapists usually ask a few specific questions about you and your feelings towards hypnosis. It will be important for him to establish that you really want to have this type of treatment. As we said, this form of hypnosis will not and cannot be administered against your will. He or she will also be interested in your previous knowledge of hypnosis and will want to find out if you have any misconceptions about it. Finally, the hypnotherapist will discuss any personal fears and apprehensions which you may feel about it. This discussion phase is essential in order to ensure that you are in the right state of relaxation to participate fully in the session. As with every other form of therapy, success depends upon your willingness to help him to help you. No treatment can ever be fully effective if you expect someone to do something to you, rather than doing it together.

The process of getting you into the hypnotic state is known as induction. There are many ways of inducing hypnosis but the most commonly used is to start with eye fixation. You are asked to stare at some object, while the hypnotherapist gradually starts to talk to you. He will then suggest that you close your eyes and just follow the various suggestions which he makes to you. He will commonly use some simple exercises to slow and regularise your breathing. At this point you are in a hypnotic state. It really is as simple as that. The hypnotherapist may proceed to ask you to do one or two things to demonstrate the depth of hypnosis. People report all sorts of different experiences while hypnotised. Many say that they felt that they could have just opened their eyes at any time and terminated the session. This does not mean that they were not hypnotised, but it does show once again that the hypnotic state is largely voluntary. You do not lose control of yourself.

While you are in the hypnotic state it is possible first to become very relaxed, then gradually to respond to more and more of the suggestions which the hypnotherapist presents to you. In particular, he or she will perhaps discuss situations which cause you anxiety and suggest that you should change your reaction to these. The remarkable thing is that suggestions of this type made during hypnosis actually have an effect on you after the session is over.

At the end of the hypnotic session, you are gradually returned to normal consciousness. There is some skill in doing this well so that you do not lose any of the positive things gained during the session. If you terminate the session too rapidly, as sometimes happens if people stop it themselves, then it is possible to lose everything that you have gained. The only areas of life which will be affected by the hypnosis will be those specifically dealt with during the session. You will not be left with any sort of unwanted effects. You might be left with so-called post-hypnotic suggestions; for instance, if in the session you dealt with your anxieties about going out in public, you may have been left with a suggestion that you would automatically start to relax if you are in a public place and begin to have anxiety symptoms. Finally, some hypnotherapists make a lot of use of autohypnosis. While hypnotised they teach you how to get into the same state while you are on your own. This approach can be very valuable for people who suffer with anxiety symptoms.

Although hypnosis is widely used in conventional medical practice, it has proved difficult to investigate in the usual scientific way. Hypnosis is a very common occurrence in daily life. If you become particularly involved in watching a television programme or film, you are probably entering a mild hypnotic state. Hypnosis covers a wide range of mental experiences, from a mild absorption in something to a deep trance state. Over the years there have been a number of attempts to define accurately the various levels of hypnosis. It is difficult to do this and most scientific work now defines hypnosis in terms of scales of susceptibility. The most susceptible people will enter a hypnotic state easily, and without an involved induction procedure, while the least susceptible need considerable preparation to enter even the earliest stages. We mentioned that in some ways hypnosis is like an early stage of sleep; there is some evidence that it is more complicated than this, but a lengthy discussion of this is beyond the scope of this book. (Again the references at the back provide more information.) What is clear is that it is possible to use hypnosis for treating a wide range of different conditions, and that it can be used to induce major physical and mental effects.

CHAPTER EIGHT

Working With the Body

We come finally to a group of different methods of working with the physical body. Yoga, Alexander therapy, chiropractice and osteopathy. Each represents a sophisticated technique which can be of great benefit in many physical disorders. We have lumped them together only for convenience. Each has been claimed to be of benefit in depression but our observations lead us to think that any effect that they may have is largely indirect. None can or should be used for treating depression on its own.

We describe them as techniques for working with the body, but this is only partially accurate.

Yoga is a very ancient system. Most people associate it with sequences of contorted postures, the so-called Hatha yoga. For the serious practitioner, this type is only used to prepare and organise the body and the mind for some of the more advanced types of yoga. There are dozens of different schools of yoga and they all consider spiritual enlightenment as their ultimate goal. In recent years, there has been a lot of research into the physical and emotional effects of yoga, and some schools use specific postures and breathing techniques for treatment. It has been alleged that yoga can benefit people with depression but there is as yet no evidence for this. What is undoubtedly true is that the regular practice of yoga has benefited some who have suffered from episodes of mild depression. It must be used though with caution and we would strongly advise against using it as a treatment on its own. People who are predisposed to depression have actually been pushed into a depressive episode by the uncontrolled use of yoga postures and yoga breathing. This should never be allowed to happen but we have seen just such a case.

Christine was an intelligent young housewife with two children, aged 9 and 7. Her husband had a good job and she had not worked since the birth of her children but now admitted to being rather bored with life. She had never had any health problems, either mental or physical. She came from a large family with whom she kept in regular touch and did a lot of voluntary work in the community. In an attempt to keep fit Christine took up Hatha yoga and went to an inexperienced teacher who held classes in the local church hall. Initially, everything went well. She rapidly became far more supple and derived a great deal of benefit from the use of yoga breathing exercises. After about six months she was doing two hours of yoga each day. It was then that the problems started. She began to feel very depressed, developed problems with sleeping and lost her appetite completely. Not surprisingly, she began to lose weight and to look unwell and unkempt. Her doctor was not able to find anything physically wrong with her and diagnosed depression. He intended to treat her with antidepressants but first suggested that she should stop doing her yoga exercises for a couple of weeks. The effect was almost instantaneous. Before the two weeks were up, she had returned to her old self and has had no recurrence of depression since that time.

This is one of only two or three problems that we have ever encountered with yoga. Most people derive benefit from doing it and it is tempting to speculate that much ill-health could be prevented by the regular practice of yoga. We mention this case to emphasise the problems which may occur if any practice is taken to extremes under uncontrolled circumstances.

Osteopathy and **chiropractice** are two similar systems of treatment which have been shown to be of great benefit for dealing with problems associated with bones, joints and ligaments. There are differences in philosophy and approach in these two systems but for our purposes they can be considered together. It is occasionally claimed that each has been successfully used to treat depression, though our observations lead us to consider that when either has had this effect it is as a result of removing some underlying painful or debilitating condition. A chronic pain in your back may well make you feel depressed, and it is no surprise that the sudden relief of the symptoms may also make you feel less depressed. We have not so far seen any patient with depression alone who responded to this form of therapy and, in common with the leaders of the osteopathic and chiropractic professions, we would not suggest that these would be an appropriate alternative form of treatment.

Alexander therapy in some ways has a similarity with the fundamental ideas of the chiropractic and osteopathic schools. It is in essence a method or re-education of posture rather than a therapy as such. The Alexander practitioner considers that many ills, including depression, are caused by the chronic maintenance of bad posture. It is said that bad posture causes the normal reflexes of the body to be inhibited; for instance, you do not move as smoothly and as effortlessly as you could. This does seem to be an important method with far-reaching consequences, but we have so far only seen it used to prevent the development of further episodes rather than treating an already established case.

All these techniques may have something to offer but we must for now reserve judgement. However, there is something to the idea that regular exercise may have an effect on mood and perhaps on more profound disturbances of emotion. People who exercise regularly have always reported that they feel particularly good afterwards. Some years ago it was shown that part of the reason for this may be that regular exercise leads to the release from the brain of the chemical endorphins — the same chemicals that we met in our discussion of the placebo response. It is these chemicals which may actually make us addicted to exercise. Based on these observations, a study was performed to look at the effect of regular exercise on a population of severely depressed people in a mental hospital. One group of the patients were asked to do regular aerobic exercise for three months. At the end of this time they were significantly less depressed than the non-exercisers. If was not a perfect scientific study but the results are still very interesting. This leads to our final conclusion, in addition to a regular, balanced diet, take some regular exercise. It should not be strenuous, unless you are already fit, but gradually increase it over a period of time.

Choosing a therapy for you

We have dealt with only a small number of the alternatives to medical treatment. There are many others, in particular herbalism and aromatherapy that are alleged to have helped some people with depression, but we have never ourselves seen these work. Even with the fairly short list which we have discussed, how do you decide which may be for you?

The first point is that all the medical alternatives insist that you take an active part in the healing process. There are people who wander from one form of therapy to another in the hope that something will be done *to* them. If this is what you want, then the alternative therapies are not for you. There are now a few clinics and practitioners who use more than one type of therapy to deal with a person, and there may be a lot of sense in this. If you have not responded to two different alternative therapies, there is probably no point in going for a third. Despite all the differences in these therapies and how they set about things, we have never yet seen someone who kept changing horses and then finally found a therapy that worked.

It is difficult for anyone to assess accurately their own degree of depression, and for this reason we suggest that if you feel that you or a friend or family member needs treatment, then they should be seen first by their own doctor. If then you decide to go for alternative therapy, you will probably find that your doctor will be interested to hear how you get on. He is unlikely to dismiss the idea. Our observations lead us to think that many of the alternative therapies do have an enormous amount to offer and can be used most effectively for the less severe and more chronic types of depression.

Most of the major schools of alternative medicine have now organised themselves so that they hold registers of fully trained practitioners. We suggest that you should only use therapists who appear on these registers. (We give details of some at the end of the book.)

Finally, which therapy? There are no hard and fast rules. If you know of a practitioner, or if a friend or colleague tells you of a reliable one, then that may be a good start. Your doctor may also know of a practitioner in whom he has confidence. We have tried to give something of the flavour of some types of alternative therapy so that you can make a more informed decision. If, despite reading that acupuncture does not hurt, you still do not like the idea of a therapy which may involve needles, then go for one of the alternatives. Similarly, if you find that the idea of using the infinitesimal doses of homoeopathy is too far-fetched, then try a different approach. Although we have seen many excellent results with the different therapies, do not expect miracles.

When you have finally made your decision, then first meet the therapist and decide if you can get on with him. Every successful practitioner, whether a doctor or alternative therapist, has also got to be a healer but you will never be able to work together if you do not have confidence in him.

CHAPTER NINE

What Causes Depression? The Latest Research

The fact that depression is so common is one reason why it has attracted so much attention from researchers. Their results have led to the rapid evolution of our ideas about the possible causes and associations of depression. A detailed review of this research is beyond the scope of this book, as is the complete presentation of current views regarding the possible causes of depression. Instead, we shall focus on a few selective areas of research, which we hope might offer the reader a flavour of this work and also of current thinking about depression. No single model alone explains our current knowledge of depression. None of the models of depression we shall describe is necessarily exclusive of the others. Indeed, one of the most intriguing aspects of our increasing knowledge of depression has been the discovery of possible links between models which have had quite different origins. For convenience, we shall divide our survey of research into three broad areas: the first deals with 'physical' or biological associations of depression; the second with social factors which are potentially important; and the third with psychological factors.

Before considering any specific research findings, it is worth stressing a few points about research into depression in general. As we have seen, 'depression' is not a unitary concept; the term defines a whole range of conditions which differ in their manifestations, severity and so on. There is no reason to believe that all forms of depression have the same cause. Equally, it is very important for researchers to define the kind of depression they are investigating, to be clear and explicit in the diagnoses they use. This allows their results to be compared with those of others who studied the same type of depression, and also indicates the relevance of their results for particular people who suffer depression. In many areas of medicine outside psychiatry, this process of discriminating between a person who has disease 'X' and someone else who does not have 'X' is helped by the use of laboratory tests. For example, the finding of excessive amounts of sugar in the blood helps to confirm the diagnosis of diabetes mellitus, the growth from sputum of the tubercle bacillus confirms the diagnosis of tuberculosis. The possibility of finding some 'biological marker' for depression, of developing a blood test, has motivated a considerable research effort into biological causes and associations of depression. As yet, however, laboratory tests have been of only limited use in psychiatry in general and in depression in particular.

The last two decades have seen the development of a number of 'operational definitions' of depression. These are like shopping lists of features of depression, a specified number of which have to be present before the researchers will consider a person 'depressed'. While this allows researchers to compare their findings more adequately, we are still left with the question — how does this help the depressed individual? It is often difficult to fit the findings of researchers or the statements in textbooks to the experiences of individuals in real life. The results of such research also allow us only to consider probabilities, to talk in terms of statistics. This reminds us that human beings are inevitably more complex than the models we devise in our attempt to understand them.

It is also worth noting that, although this section is concerned with the causes of depression, it is often difficult to distinguish *causes* from *associations*. Because one discovers an association between A and B, this does not necessarily mean that A caused B, or, for that matter, that B caused A. While some of the factors we shall describe which are associated with depression may indeed turn out to be causes, future research is likely to show that other factors result from depression. We refer to all of these as 'causes' only for the sake of simplicity.

Physical causes

Genetics and the inheritance of depression

That depression may sometimes be inherited is one of the major pieces of evidence favouring a biological component in its causation.

Depression sometimes runs in families. Although the pattern of its transmission from one generation to the next fits with it being an inherited disorder, the same pattern may be explained in other ways. For example, there is good evidence that being brought up by a depressed parent may have a considerable effect on a child. So the family environment may play an important role in the 'handing down' of depression from parents to children. This is the dilemma, well recognised in such research, of distinguishing 'nature' from 'nurture'. However, better evidence of a genetic component in depression comes from two other sources: studies of twins, and studies of people who have been adopted.

Identical twins share exactly the same genes, they have the same genetic make-up; non-identical twins do not have exactly the same genetic make-up, but share as many common genes as would brothers or sisters. If one twin possesses genes that somehow code for depression, then the chances of the other twin possessing the same genes are clearly greater if the twins are identical than when they are non-identical. By contrast, if there is no genetic influence at work, there is little reason to believe that the occurrence of depression should be any different comparing identical with non-identical twins. Three observations are important here: first, twins are no more or less likely than anyone else to develop depression, thus being a twin does not in itself predispose to depression; the second observation is that, if one twin has a history of depression, the chances of the second twin becoming depressed at some stage are very much higher if the twins are identical, which supports the existence of a genetic component to depression; furthermore, the same applies even if the twins are raised apart from each other, which should minimise the environmental influences they share.

The adoption studies have concerned people who were separated from their parents and adopted at an early age.

Regardless of the adoptive parents, people whose natural parents have a history of depression are more likely to suffer depression themselves than others of the same age and sex who were adopted away at a similar age but born to parents without any history of depression. This again supports the importance of a genetic component in depression.

Studies such as these have indicated that the genetic influence is strongest when people have manic depressive illness (also called bipolar affective disorder — see Chapter One) and is greater for people who have psychotic depression compared to those with neurotic depression. The nature of the genetic link — whether it could be due to a single gene or more than one, for example — remains controversial.

Sex and hormones

Between the ages of 15 and 50, depression is twice as common in women as in men. Many mechanisms have been proposed to account for this difference. We shall consider some of the social and psychological explanations later in this chapter. Of the biological mechanisms that have been proposed, the effects of hormones have attracted considerable attention.

Depression after childbirth is well recognised. Some women become mildly depressed, experiencing what is commonly termed 'baby blues' or 'the blues'. This is very common — it affects about 50 per cent of all mothers. Less frequently, severe depression may follow childbirth and when this happens it follows a characteristic pattern. Usually, all is well until somewhere between the fourth and seventh post-natal day, when the mother becomes profoundly depressed and often very distressed and disturbed. This so-called post-natal psychosis follows a pattern that is sometimes different from other forms of depression but is clearly linked in some way with these other forms. For example, the close relatives of women who suffer post-natal psychoses are much more likely than expected to suffer from depression themselves.

A variety of causes have been proposed for these severe depressions following childbirth. They might be related to the 'event' of giving birth (the relationship between life events and depression will be considered in more detail later.) However, this and other psychological or social explanations are inadequate because women who miscarry or have terminations of pregnancy (both stressful events) do not show this higher risk of severe depression, neither do new fathers, who are exposed to at least some of the stresses associated with their partner giving birth. All this points to a 'biological' explanation. Post-natal psychoses start at just the time that there are very marked changes in the levels of two kinds of hormones, oestrogen and progesterone. Some researchers have suggested that it is these very rapid changes in hormone concentrations in the blood following labour which precipitate the depression in women who are particularly sensitive to such changes. Others have suggested that the main influence is due to the changing concentration of salts in the blood or the changing amount of water retained in the body. As yet, no convincing and consistent differences have been found in any of these factors when comparing women who develop post-natal psychoses with those who do not. This would suggest that, whatever changes are important, they only give rise to the depression in women who are susceptible for another reason, for example genetically.

Even though we do not adequately understand what causes post-natal psychoses, their existence is well established and not disputed. The same cannot be said of premenstrual depression. Examination of most of the older research studies has revealed flaws in their methods and problems with their conclusions. More recent work, which has paid close attention to detail, suggests that premenstrual symptoms do not themselves cause depression or other symptoms, but tend to worsen such features of depression as are already present. As for the post-natal psychoses, hormonal changes during menstruation have been implicated in this, as has water retention. However, neither of these single factors alone can account for the association between depression and premenstrual symptoms. Similarly, a simple explanation is unlikely to emerge for the fact that some women who take oral contraceptives also become depressed, although the hormones that go to make up the pill undoubtedly play a role here.

Brain biochemistry and depression

The discussion of the effects of sex hormones on brain function leads us quite naturally to one of the most fascinating areas of modern medical science. It is the bridge between the biological chemistry of the brain itself and the human mind. Every year now brings a vast amount of new research information, much of it in such rarefied areas that only a few scientists can hope to understand everything that is being achieved. But amidst this avalanche of information, a number of crucial new principles are beginning to emerge. It is no longer far-fetched to speculate that we are now living in the age during which most of the major mental illnesses will be understood in a way that will make treatment both reliable and safe. However, it is the opinion of the authors that even when we reach that stage, there will still be a great need both to understand and to deal with the whole person. The chemical breakthroughs will if anything amplify the need to deal with the individual. Biochemistry will not provide all the answers.

Much of the research data concerning the biological basis of depression has been obtained by a combination of inference based on the mode of action of drugs which are useful in depression, and from some animal studies. It is still not possible to study the brain directly in humans, although two new pieces of scientific equipment make it possible that we may soon be able to do so. These are two types of scanner, one known as the magnetic resonance scanner and the other known as the positron emission tomographic scanner (PET scanner). It now looks very much as if the changes in brain function which accompany depression are quite different in each of the different types of depression. This was why we commented right at the beginning of this chapter about the difficulty in interpreting some particular pieces of research in which the distinctions between different types of depression have not been made clear.

The story of the development of ideas concerning brain biochemistry and depression has been a wonderful piece of detective work. A few clues were picked up, and from these a picture is now emerging. The first clues as to the nature of the chemical changes in the brain of the depressed person came from a consideration of some of the physical and mental symptoms of depression. In the section on the clinical features of depression we commented on three very common types of symptom –

anorexia or loss of appetite, which may lead to sometimes profound weight loss, sleep disturbance, and loss of libido or sex drive. Over the last ten years or so, a great deal of research has been done which tells us something about how the normal functions of eating, sleeping and the sex drive come about. Each is a very basic drive and underlies a good deal of our behaviour. Furthermore, there are many major similarities between the way in which each of these drives occurs in animals and in humans.

In severe depression, at least 60 per cent of patients reduce their food intake. Many say that they do not feel like eating and others complain that food ceases to interest them and may even become tasteless. It seems that in severe depression people suffer a generalised loss of gratification in performing most activities — nothing appears rewarding, including those activities normally associated with powerful biological drives such as eating and sex. In some cases it may just be that appetite is lost because of reduced physical activity, another common feature of depression. It is not difficult to imagine some other reasons for this loss of drive, but quite recently it was decided that it might be worth looking at the neurology of these effects — which sites in the brain might be responsible for them. It has been known for some time that the main parts of the brain responsible for hunger and the regulation of food intake are located in a region known as the hypothalamus, which lies very deep down in the base of the brain. There are two so-called centres, one of which tells us to eat and the other tells us when we have had enough. Normally these two centres are perfectly balanced, and only respond to cues from the body, so that smells, an empty stomach and low blood sugar make us want to eat, while a full stomach usually makes us want to stop. There are a whole host of other stimuli involved, but the crucial thing is that in depression this fundamental balance is disturbed. The key observation, as far as we are concerned here, is that there is a specific chemical system in the brain which is intimately involved in maintaining the balance between the two feeding areas in the hypothalamus of the human brain. This system relies upon a compound known as noradrenaline or norepinephrine. As we shall see, this is one of three related compounds which is now thought to have a fundamental role in at least some forms of depression.

For our next clue, we turn to the second of the symptoms of depression we mentioned above, the loss of libido which occurs in at least 60 per cent of patients with severe depression. It is not difficult to see how this in itself can lead to a vicious circle, in which lack of sex drive can lead to more depression which makes the loss of libido worse still, and so on. Human sexual functions are extremely complex and many are controlled or at the least modulated by a group of hormones which are normally secreted by the anterior pituitary gland, situated just below the hypothalamus which is involved in feeding behaviour. This same organ, the hypothalamus, is responsible for controlling the secretion of these sex hormones. The way in which it does this is via a sequence of chemical compounds, which include noradrenaline and another of the three chemicals thought to be involved in depression — dopamine. There is now some very strong evidence to suggest that the loss of libido in depression, and perhaps also one other symptom, namely impotence, are caused directly by chemical and hormonal imbalances in this portion of the brain.

So now we have the hint that two chemical compounds are involved in the symptoms of depression. There is, however, a third: this is the compound known as serotonin or 5-hydroxytryptamine. It is only in recent years that much has been learned about the effects of this substance in the brain. But it turns out that it is intimately involved in a number of crucial functions in the brain and in behaviour. The first suggestion that it might be concerned in depression came from a consideration of the third of our symptoms — sleep disturbance. It is only now becoming clear that serotonin is one of the most important of the brain chemicals controlling sleep. While it is found all over the brain in varying amounts, there are particularly large quantities of it in the area known as the brain stem. It is here that much of the control of sleep occurs. Very recently, it has also been discovered that serotonin has a major role in the way in which we perceive pain. This may be most important in depression — the complaints of many depressed people suggest that they experience an alteration in pain sensitivity. Even in mild depression, minor physical symptoms may seem intolerable, and although there may be straightforward psychological reasons for this, it is intriguing to speculate that this symptom too may be caused by a chemical imbalance in the brain.

These then are the clues which seem to indicate an unholy trinity of chemicals involved in depression — noradrenaline, dopamine and serotonin.

It is now some twenty years since it was proposed that some forms of severe depression may be caused by a chemical imbalance in some part of the brain's biochemistry. When it was first proposed, there was really very little known about the brain effects of dopamine and serotonin, but as more has been discovered the basic concept has been able to evolve to take in many, but not yet all, of the facts as they have emerged.

All this suggests that a chemical imbalance may be a crucial event in depression. But is there any proof that it is important? Well, the answer to this is yes. Much of the recent research data has come from a study of the effects of drugs used in treating depression. From laboratory experiments, much has been learnt concerning the ways in which these drugs have their action. Virtually all antidepressants have a major action in one or more of our three chemical systems. That in itself is not proof positive that one or other of these chemicals is the actual cause of depression, especially since most drugs have more than one action, but taken altogether the evidence in favour of this hypothesis is becoming very strong. Despite this, this hypothesis, like any other, will have to continue to evolve as more is discovered, and eventually it may need to be replaced by something new. That is the way things always work in science — we have never completely finished!

Whatever the future may hold for this theory as to the possible causes of depression, it has already proved to be immensely valuable. Within the last few years the first of a new range of tailor-made antidepressants have become available. Drugs which aim deliberately to restore balance in the serotonin system have already proved their worth, and more of these new, and hopefully safer and more reliable, drugs are on their way at this moment.

This does still leave us with a major problem. What is it that causes this biochemical disturbance in the first place? We know that such a derangement in the three chemical systems will cause symptoms of depression in some animals, and certain drugs which interfere with these systems in humans may cause depression as a side-effect. We know also that the important parts of the brain in depression are the hypothalamus and its surrounding areas. But still it is not clear why the changes we have mentioned appear to occur spontaneously in humans at the onset of a depressive episode. For this reason there is now a considerable research effort directed towards examining people before they become depressed to see whether any common factors can be determined. The people who are being studied most carefully are those who appear to be particularly vulnerable to becoming depressed; that is, people who have a strong family history of depression or of some other behavioural disorder, and people who have a certain biochemical make-up which may predispose them to depression.

It has been known for some time that severely depressed people have a range of hormonal imbalances. We have already referred to disturbances in sex hormones but it transpires that there are others. There are at least fifty different hormones in the body and more are being discovered all the time. It now appears that there are disturbances in most if not all the hormones which come from the hypothalamus and the pituitary gland. Disturbances here have effects on many other glands in the body, but in particular on the adrenal glands which are situated just above the kidneys. The adrenal glands are responsible for producing some of the so-called 'stress hormones' — adrenaline, noradrenaline (which also occurs in the brain) and cortisol.

It is the last of these, cortisol, which has attracted a great deal of attention. When we are healthy, the concentration of cortisol in the blood does not remain constant. The amount released into the bloodstream fluctuates in a characteristic way depending on the time of day. Also, its release into the blood can be suppressed by a drug called dexamethasone; this is the basis of the dexamethasone suppression test. In a majority of patients with endogenous depression, the amount of cortisol in their blood is higher than expected and dexamethasone fails to suppress its secretion. Furthermore, as the depression is treated these odd results no longer occur, they go back to normal. For many years it was thought that this was such a non-specific test that it was of little use. It was often found to be abnormal in alcoholism or even just during illness generally. It now seems, though, that there are ways of using the test which may make it possible to predict the people at a particular risk of developing depression, and these people can be watched and perhaps studied in more detail. Considerably more work is needed before we can say whether this test may have any use in individual patients, but it represents a most important attempt to learn something about the causes of depression.

It is relevant to ask why only some patients show this change in the metabolism of the hormone cortisol. The reason is that within all our medical diagnostic groups there are different types of depression. Much of the research effort of the last few years has been geared towards getting a better idea about what makes different people with depression behave and respond in such different ways.

Part of the answer to our question about what actually causes the chemical changes in the brain may be related to the way in which the different chemical systems and the hormonal systems interact in the brains of individual people. We mentioned earlier that there are as many as fifty different hormones in the body. During the last ten years it has become clear that many of these same hormones are present in the brain, and here they have major functions that are only now being discovered. Many of these functions relate to those same drives and inhibitions that we know occur in depression. The old model of three chemicals will need to be expanded to include perhaps thirty or forty. It might seem that this will present an impossible problem to tackle within anyone's lifetime. Paradoxically, it may well be that this very complexity gives us some clues as to the basic functioning of parts of the brain and how these may go wrong. One way of looking at the normal brain, and how it may go wrong in depression, is to view the brain as a system which is normally balanced and carefully organised. If one part of the system goes wrong then the whole balance is disturbed to some extent but for the most part the rest of the system can compensate. But, if a key area is affected, or if more than one part goes wrong at a time, then the attempts of the whole system to compensate will become more and more difficult. Eventually the system breaks down and depression may be the consequence. Imagine riding on a bicycle: once you have learnt how, it is relatively easy to keep your balance. There are a series of feedbacks that keep you upright. You can even keep your balance if there is a strong cross-wind, but if at the same time you get a flat tyre and the road is wet, it is highly likely that you will fall. It is very likely that a similar group of things going wrong like this in the brain may trigger off depression. We do not know whether it is possible to learn to avoid depression in the same way that you can learn to ride a bicycle, but there is some preliminary evidence to suggest that some people do indeed manage to avoid depression altogether, even when their genes and their circumstances should cause it to happen.

What could be the equivalent of a strong cross-wind, a flat tyre and a wet road in the human brain? Well, we shall in a moment be discussing some of the recent research findings concerning the role of psychological and social factors in the causation of depression. It is worth mentioning at this point that anything which occurs in the outside world is reflected by changes occurring in the brain. As you read this page, your eyes make very rapid scanning movements of the printed words and the visual images are transmitted to the back part of your brain which starts the process of decoding the information, helping you to relate this information to facts which you know already. This initiates the process of understanding what you are reading. It is a highly active sequence of events and your brain is never quite the same again. Subtle chemical changes have been started which ultimately affect the whole of your brain. Now, if instead of reading this book, something unsettling happens, a burglary or a bereavement perhaps, then again chemical changes occur in the brain and can start to disturb your normal equilibrium. This is the cross-wind. If it then happens that this unsettling event ocurrs to someone whose balance has already been disturbed, perhaps by genetic make-up, or hormones, or past experience, then you may have the equivalent of the flat tyre and the wet road. We all know people who have the most dreadful things happen to them and yet never seem to turn a hair. We tend to call them well balanced, or sometimes we see them as being perhaps a bit dull, but it is probably quite true that many of these people do literally have brains that respond less than others to things in the environment or in themselves. This does not make them dull or insensitive and more than just demonstrating another major difference between people, it illustrates the likely complexity of the factors accounting for such differences.

It is often said that a certain mild lack of mental balance is one of the things which gives us our drives, our ambitions and makes us more imaginative. Some have then gone on to say that we should therefore not consider ever treating or helping people with depression, since any form of treatment might interfere with these positive parts of the personality. The evidence for this is supposed to be that many great creative geniuses like Isaac Newton, Goethe and Samuel Jonson all suffered from episodes of depression, sometimes alternating with quite manic episodes. So did these people have some imbalance of brain chemistry which both caused depression and their genius? Well, it would be a nice idea but it is almost certainly not true. Some years ago a study was performed to look at the incidence of mental disorder amongst a large group of British male geniuses, and the results showed that depression was no more common among the members of this group than it was in the rest of the population. There is no doubt that some of the older forms of treatment for depression did sometimes lead to a blunting of parts of the personality, but that is precisely the reason that so much research continues in depression, to find ways of helping people which do not have these unwanted side-effects — and we are already coming close to achieving this goal.

Physical illness as a cause of depression

Although it now seems that depression usually occurs as a consequence of several things conspiring together, we have said already that people with a particularly strong family history are more prone than others to develop certain types of depression. It would seem that a heavy dose of one risk factor can outweigh any amount of innate chemical balance in the brain. To continue with our bicycle analogy, one very strong gust of wind may knock us off the bicycle, even on a dry road with our tyres in perfectly good condition.

Apart from genetic risk factors, what other things may do this? Well, there are a great many physical illnesses which may cause depression as a prominent part of their symptomatology. Sometimes the depression may be so prominent that it is the first thing people complain of, never imagining that it has been caused by some underlying illness. With some diseases, it is easy to imagine that depression might occur. Cancer, chronic pain, heart disease, and even some less chronic but nonetheless painful or debilitating diseases may lead to depression. Most doctors are only too well aware of this element of an illness, and although ultimately the most satisfactory way of dealing with this type of depression is to treat the underlying disorder, this is not always possible. One very important element of the depression which may accompany some other disease, is that a vicious circle may be set up in which depression makes the symptoms worse, which in turn makes the depression worse, and so it goes on. It is often with these patients that the highest levels of skill are required in treatment. We shall discuss this in a little more detail further on.

Apart from such diseases, there are a number of others in which depression may become a major feature. Perhaps the most tantalising and also the most difficult to treat are viral infections, many of which are regularly complicated by depression. There is now very strong evidence that in many viral infections depression is caused directly by the infection, rather than just being a consequence of feeling unwell. To this day we do not know the identities of all the viruses which may cause these symptoms, but the more efforts that are made to discover whether depressed people have been exposed to viruses, the more are found. It is important to stress that just because we find evidence of a past infection in a depressed person, in no way does this mean that the virus was necessarily responsible. We have all had many viral infections but it is only a very few which cause depression as a long-term problem. We would normally only consider that a virus was responsible if somebody who has never before had depression or any other mental disorder suddenly develops it in association with clear evidence of an infection. Sometimes the depression is out of all proportion to the severity of the infection and it becomes necessary to probe hard.

The classical infection which may lead to depression is glandular fever. Typically this is caused by one type of virus but it can produce a whole range of symptoms. The particular symptoms which somebody may get are probably determined by quite a number of factors, including the sub-type of the virus and one's general state of health and well-being. After many of the first symptoms of glandular fever have settled, the depression may go on for a very long time. Some people shrug off the virus and the depression very rapidly but for others the depression may go on for a year or more and require intensive treatment, not of the infection but of the depression itself. It is still difficult to be certain why this should be but some very recent research may at last reveal the answer. It is well known that the immune system comes into play during viral infections as part of the body's response to infection. What is generally far less well known is that in addition to the normal immune reactions, viruses cause many of the cells of the body to produce a class of proteins which are designed to prevent further viral infection. Several of these have been discovered and collectively they are known as the interferons. Very recently, some of these interferons have been synthesised and they are now undergoing trials in a number of clinical conditions to see if they can be used in treatment. What is so interesting is that at least one of them, when administered to humans regularly, causes a brief episode of euphoria after which many people become profoundly depressed. Putting these facts together, it now seems highly likely that at least a part of the depression which may be caused by viral infections is a result of these interferons produced by the viruses which are infecting some of the cells of the body.

There is, however, one other important piece of research which may have a bearing on the depression caused by viruses. One of the most modern and sophisticated pieces of scientific equipment which is being brought to bear on medical problems is the magnetic resonance scanner, which we mentioned earlier. It is possible to use this tool to study certain elements of the metabolism of the body without doing anything damaging or invasive. The technical details do not concern us here, but already magnetic resonance is revolutionising many areas of science and medicine. Recently a patient who had suffered with chronic exhaustion and depression ever since a viral infection four years earlier was investigated using this technique. The metabolism in the muscles of his forearm was studied in great detail and it was found that there was a major abnormality of a highly unusual type. In most of us, our metabolism is closely linked to the requirements of our bodies but in this man the normal linkage was disturbed, with the consequence that his metabolism could just not cope with any changes, so in effect he could never get his muscle metabolism out of first gear. We must await further research, but already it seems possible that these findings will have a direct bearing on the depression which may follow infections with many different viruses.

It has been known for many years that diseases of several different hormone-producing glands may cause depression. The ones most often talked about are diseases of the thyroid gland and occasionally those of the adrenal glands. It has also been suggested that there may be a higher than average incidence of depression in diabetes mellitus, so-called sugar diabetes. For a long time it was by no means certain why this should be; there was a good deal of speculation but no hard facts. Now it turns out that the thyroid hormones are intimately involved in the control of the metabolism of the brain, and in particular in the manufacture and action of several of the chemicals in the brain itself. And as it happens, they have major actions on the three key chemicals which we discussed earlier, noradrenaline, serotonin and dopamine. With thyroid disease, it is normally underactivity of the gland which is associated with depression and this induces major imbalances in the relationships between these three chemicals. Similarly, several of the hormones produced by the adrenal gland have important functions in maintaining a healthy equilibrium between the chemical systems of the brain.

A difficult but interesting problem is whether or not depression is commoner in people with diabetes; difficult not only because the research findings are variable, but also because there are many possible factors which might contribute to depression among diabetics. However, the factor which concerns us here is the basic problem underlying diabetes itself, namely a lack of, or a resistance to, the hormone insulin. There are many functions of insulin but a key one is its control of the entry of glucose into many of the cells of the body. This does not occur normally in diabetics, and so without a diet or some other form of treatment they tend to run a high blood sugar level. The point of importance to us here is that in very many diabetics the basic problem is not that they have a deficiency of the hormone insulin, but that the cells of their bodies are resistant to the action of insulin. As a result they have very high circulating levels of the hormone. Now, it has recently been discovered that insulin has some very specific actions on the absorption into the brain of certain amino acids. The amino acids are the basic building blocks of proteins, but they are also the compounds from which our three key brain chemicals are manufactured. Thus one contributing factor to depression in diabetes could be the altered absorption of amino acids into the brain under the influence of abnormally high levels of insulin.

One of these amino acids is called tryptophan and it is from this that serotonin is made. It has been shown that if healthy volunteers are given even a single dose of tryptophan, they become tired, lethargic and depressed in a matter of hours. This almost certainly happens because of a rise in the manufacture of serotonin in the brain. This effect only occurs after taking a single dose of tryptophan. If tryptophan is taken continuously, it appears to have the opposite effect — there is some evidence that it enhances the action of the tricyclic antidepressants and may even have some antidepressant effects in its own right. The key thing is the length of exposure to the substance.

It has recently been discovered that eating a meal containing a lot of carbohydrate but not much protein will, at least in animals, raise the levels of tryptophan and serotonin in the brain. This is probably the reason why we usually tend to feel lethargic after a high carbohydrate meal. Now it turns out that carbohydrates do this by increasing the secretion of insulin, which in turn increases the absorption of tryptophan by the brain. As we said just now, in many diabetics there are high levels of insulin in the blood and the conditions should be just right for depression to occur. It is remarkable that not more of them have depression, and maybe this confirms the idea that the brain has an amazing ability to keep itself in balance, so long as not too many things go wrong at once and it has time to recover from attack.

The physical consequences of depression

A number of the symptoms of depression which we described in the first section of this book are related to disturbances of various hormones, coupled with disturbances in the chemical systems of the brain itself. As we have already noted, these include loss of the sex drive, loss of appetite and disturbance of normal sleep rhythm. But there are other physical consequences of depression that we can now understand.

A disturbance in the balance of the three basic brain chemicals leads to a generalised slowing of many of the functions of the body. Depressed people often appear slow in their movements, their thinking slows, and they may become constipated. The systems of the brain responsible for these functions all depend on a normal balance between this group of chemicals and a disturbance of one or more of them is reflected in the physical and mental slowing.

What has only recently been discovered is that depression is associated with profound disturbances in the normal functioning of the immune system. It has now been suggested that depressive illnesses are associated with an increased risk of infection, cancer, and the so-called autoimmune diseases in which the body's own immune system starts attacking its own cells. It has now been shown quite clearly that in depression the normal defences based on the white cells of the blood just cease to function efficiently. This is partly a consequence of the high level of the hormone cortisol which is found in some types of depression, but in the last two years it has been shown that another factor is the levels in the blood of the chemicals known as endorphins. These are the same chemicals that we met earlier in our discussion of placebo reactions. But it now seems that in many depressed people there are abnormalities in endorphins which suppress the normal functioning of the immune system.

This phenomenon has been examined in more detail in bereavement which, as we saw in Chapter One, is in some ways similar to depression. It has been known throughout history that people have a very high risk of dying in the first six months after the death of their husband or wife, and the risk is particularly high for men. One of the main reasons for this again is a reduction in the efficiency of the immune system, caused by changes in hormonal levels, but probably also by some other factors which are not yet understood. This knowledge is more than just idle curiosity, it shows yet again that there are many, many reasons for trying to understand and treat depression — left alone it can cause more than just misery for the individual and his family.

Social factors

Sex differences in depression

Researchers from many different countries have concluded that depression is more common among women than men. We have already seen that certain hormonal changes to which women are subject offer one reason for this sex difference in the occurrence of depression. However, this is unlikely to be the complete answer and numerous other explanations have been proposed. For example, it has been suggested that women tend to visit their doctors more frequently than men, and also to discuss distress and other 'psychological' symptoms more openly with doctors and other professionals, as well as with friends. Another suggestion is that under circumstances in which women become depressed, their male relatives might turn to alcohol. However, as with all research in this field, it has proved very difficult to distinguish *effects* from *causes*. Excessive use of alcohol may be the result of depression or its cause. Having a close relative who drinks excessively may itself be a sufficient cause for depression.

Explanations for sex differences in the occurrence of depression must also account for the observation that, for women, marriage tends to increase their chances of developing depression, while the opposite happens for men — married men suffer depression less frequently than those who are single or separated. This has given rise to considerable speculation, much of it focused on the demeaning influence of being 'a housewife' on a woman's social status. Broader feminine stereotypes have also been suggested to contribute to the greater frequency of depression in women. Feminists argue that women have difficulty freeing themselves from such stereotypes because these tend to be publicly reinforced by doctors and others. It is interesting that, while women are much more likely than men to be diagnosed and treated for depression, men and women do not differ significantly in the frequency or nature of the depressive symptoms they show during bereavement. As we noted in Chapter One, depression during bereavement is usually regarded as 'normal' and adaptive. The current development of psychological models of depression with a feminist perspective should contribute to our understanding of this issue. Such models are also likely to suggest particular questions which can be addressed in future research.

Life events and vulnerability to depression

The work of Professor George Brown and his colleagues provides a very good example of research into the social origins of depression. For a variety of reasons, most of this research has concentrated on depression in women — less is understood of the social components of depression in men. Several researchers, including George Brown himself, have found that individuals who become depressed are more likely than others to have recently suffered a threatening event in their lives. Such 'life events' are difficult to investigate and controversy still surrounds their precise definition and meaning. Not all life events, even when they are considered severe, predispose to depression. Also, the problem again arises of distinguishing cause from effect. For example, a relationship may end because one partner becomes depressed, or the ending of the relationship might lead to depression. Thus researchers have needed to give much thought to which life events they should include in their investigations and which should be discounted.

Even when life events have been rigorously defined, the link between these and depression is complex. For example, working-class women tend to experience more frequent and severe life events than their middle-class counterparts. Superficially, this might be thought to account for the increased occurrence of depression in working-class women relative to others. However, there is an additional factor. Even when faced with similarly threatening life events, middle-class women are less likely than working-class women to develop depression. To account for such observations, Brown and his colleagues suggested that the effects of life events on depression are mediated by what they called 'vulnerability factors'. Certain life events predispose to depression only in the presence of certain vulnerability factors, which happen to occur more frequently among working-class women than among others. Based on their work in London, Brown and Harris proposed four such vulnerability factors applying to women: the lack of a confiding relationship with a spouse or similar partner; the presence at home of three or more children under the age of 14 years; the lack of employment outside the home; and separation from one's mother before the age of 11 years.

The last of these vulnerability factors is different from the others because it relates not to the present but to the past. Separation from the mother at an early age also proved interesting for another reason. The researchers noted that the depressed women in their study whose mothers had *died* tended to show features of depression which were different from those of women who had been separated from their mothers for other reasons, for example, by the divorce of their parents. However, all other things being equal, a women whose mother died when she was very young was no more likely to become depressed following a life event than another woman whose separation from her mother had a different cause. In other words, while *any* form of separation from mother at an early age increased the chances of a woman becoming depressed after a significant life event, the nature of that separation influenced the kind of depression the person suffered. Brown and his colleagues described early separation from the mother as a 'symptom-formation factor'. Thus vulnerability factors affect the *risk* of someone becoming depressed after an adverse life event, while symptom-formation factors influence the *form* of the depression if it develops. We shall return to the issue of early separation from one's mother later.

Brown and his colleagues have applied that same model of depression in other communities they have studied, notably in the rural setting of the Hebrides in Scotland. There, threatening life events were less frequent than in London and depression also occurred less frequently. Not surprisingly, the vulnerability factors found among London women were inappropriate in the Hebrides. In the Hebrides, not going to church regularly emerged as a vulnerability factor, as did departure from the traditional lifestyle of crofting and fishing. Women who lived in council houses were more likely to develop depression than those who retained the traditional way of life. As in the London study, factors were found that did not increase the risk of depression but influenced its nature. For example, of the women who became depressed following the death of a close relative, those who were not married took longer to recover than the married women. Furthermore, among this group of unmarried women, those who were widowed or divorced tended to suffer symptoms which were different from those of the women who had never married.

This model, linking life events (or 'provoking factors') with depression via vulnerability factors, is widely quoted and has had considerable influence on current thinking about the social origins of depression. The work of Brown and his colleagues has been repeated by other researchers in different parts of Britain and elsewhere. The basic model seems to be widely applicable although the details differ depending on the setting. For example, the vulnerability factors described above were different in London and in the Hebrides. Another study from Calgary in Canada has suggested that the vulnerability factors there may be different from those found in London. In a sense, this is hardly surprising; vulnerability factors may be seen as measures of social support (or the lack of it), and the support available is likely to vary from one community to another. Critics of the model have suggested that its authors have gone further in their conclusions about the social origins of depression than the information so far collected allows. Nevertheless, this work continues to act as an important stimulus for further research and debate.

Life events and difficulties may seem very remote from the

biochemical and hormonal changes in depression which we discussed earlier in this section. However, researchers have begun to discover some tantalising links here. We mentioned above that the hormone cortisol is among those which show changes in depression. A very recent study compared what happened to cortisol levels in two groups of depressed people, those who had suffered a recent severe life event before the start of their depression and those whose depression was not preceded by such an event. The results suggested that abnormally high cortisol levels were more likely in the group whose depression followed a severe life event.

Unemployment

Another area of active research relates to the potential effects on mental health of unemployment. The suicide rate is higher among the unemployed than among those in paid employment. The unemployed are also over-represented among admissions to hospital following deliberate overdoses of drugs and other forms of deliberate self-harm. A recent study from Edinburgh showed that deliberate self-harm was at least ten times more frequent among unemployed men than among their employed counterparts. Furthermore, the rise in the frequency of deliberate self-harm coincided with the rise in the number of men out of work. Although there is only a weak relationship between deliberate self-harm and depression, such data emphasise the considerable impact of unemployment on mental health in general.

Among school-leavers, those who fail to find employment suffer more symptoms like sleep disturbance, anxiety and feelings of depression than those who manage to find work. However, this result could mean either that those out of work become unwell, or that those who start off unwell are less successful at finding work. The researchers in this particular study first screened their subjects (more than 1,000 British 16-year olds) before they left school, and no differences were found in mental health between those who subsequently became unemployed after leaving school and those who succeeded in finding a job. Thus it appears that the failure to find work leads to a deterioration in mental health, often with symptoms of depression. Furthermore, such symptoms of mental distress fell sharply when those who had been unemployed managed to find a job. Another recent piece of research involved a group of journalists who faced the threat of redundancy. While facing redundancy, more than one-third of the journalists had symptoms like poor sleep, fatigue and feelings of depression. A sizeable proportion of this group with symptoms recovered when the redundancy notices were withdrawn.

The effects of unemployment on mental health in general and on depression in particular are mediated by a number of other factors. For example, in terms of its effects on mental health, unemployment tends to have a greater effect on the middle-aged compared with younger or older people. Also, the more we want a job (and the greater the pressure from others to find a job), the more our mental health is likely to suffer during unemployment. If we have someone to turn to for help with money, or someone to suggest interesting things to do (both examples of *practical* support), this tends to protect us against the harmful effects of being without work. By contrast, *emotional* support appears to have little effect here. More research, leading to better understanding of such factors, will be necessary if we are to limit the health hazards of unemployment. However, it is worth noting also that a minority of people report an improvement in their mental health when they are without work. Some of us feel better having given up very stressful jobs, while others manage to make a positive adjustment to their increased leisure time.

Psychological factors

Learned helplessness

Of the behavioural models of depression, that of 'learned helplessness' is probably the best known. This concept is based on work with animals; for example, a dog is subjected to repeated unpleasant stimuli (like shocks) while at the same time being restrained (in a harness, for example) from taking action to avoid the stimuli. When the dog is unharnessed and thus given the opportunity to evade the unpleasant stimuli, it nevertheless remains still and continues to suffer them. This is an example of 'learned helplessness'. It can be reversed by actively moving the animal away from the unpleasant stimulus. There has also been some suggestion that tricyclic antidepressants may be effective in reversing this type of behaviour. It was suggested that this situation parallels depression in humans because, in both cases, the individual feels he has lost his usual control over his environment and therefore feels 'hopeless' and 'helpless'. In other words, the individual has attributed certain characteristics to himself and to the situation around him. This process of attribution is important in helping all of us to explain the behaviour of others around us. It has given rise to attribution theory, which deals with the rules people use to interpret the behaviour of others. The learned helplessness model has recently been reformulated in terms of attribution theory — the depressed person sees everything beyond his control and makes other errors of attribution. This is referred to as a 'maladaptive attributional style'.

The cognitive model of depression

Although the concept of learned helplessness sounds very plausible and has attracted much attention, its relevance to clinical depression remains questionable. By contrast, the cognitive theory of depression is widely accepted as very important and is relevant to the treatment of depression, as we saw in Chapter Two. Superficially, this may appear to resemble the attributional model described above. The distinctions between these models are of more concern to researchers than they need be for ourselves. The name most widely associated with the cognitive theory of depression is that of Aaron Beck, an American psychiatrist and psychotherapist. Unlike the learned helplessness model which originated from observations of experimental animals, it was Beck's work with depressed people which led him to formulate his ideas about cognitive theory.

The term 'cognition' describes a person's thoughts and the ways they are dealt with by the mind; it covers beliefs, interpretations, expectations and other aspects of thinking. Such cognitions form a link between our experiences and the way we react to them emotionally. We use cognitions to interpret our immediate experiences. Between each external event and our emotional response to it, there is a thought. Although such thoughts occur within our conscious minds, they tend to happen automatically and we are usually not aware of them in the same way that, for example, we are usually unaware of the complex bodily co-ordination involved in riding a bicycle. The same experience might evoke very different emotions in different people, depending on their cognitions. If a number of people are waiting in a queue, some might tolerate another person who tries to jump the queue, while others might have the immediate urge to forcibly eject the queue-jumper. Through past experience, each of us builds up a particular cognitive 'style', an individual repertoire of thoughts and ways of dealing with them. The theory also suggests that we all organise our cognitions into particular frameworks or packages, described as 'schemata'. These usually change with age and maturity, so that as we get older, our primitive childhood schemata are replaced by other more mature frameworks. However, it is suggested that our immature schemata are not lost for ever but merely remain dormant, sometimes re-emerging when we come under stress.

The reader may be puzzled by the difference between the abnormal cognitions to which we have just referred and delusions, which we noted in Chapter One were characteristic features of psychotic depression. For our present purpose, the important difference is that, if we become or are made aware that our automatic thoughts are abnormal, we usually have no difficulty accepting this and can then start modifying these thoughts accordingly. By contrast, someone who has a delusion will resolutely stick to it, however persuasive the arguments against it. Our cognitions usually represent a genuine attempt to link what goes on around us with the way we feel and act, whereas delusions are beliefs which may happen totally independently of everything else.

Cognitive theory holds that depression is associated with a group of maladaptive or unhelpful thoughts, which lead to what Beck has called the 'negative cognitive triad', made up of a negative view of oneself, of the world and of the future. In depression, cognitions all tend to become negative and distorted. The depressed person is not aware of this happening because like everyone else he takes for granted that his automatic thoughts are true. One component of cognitive therapy involves training the individual to become more aware of his abnormal cognitions and then to compare these with what is actually happening around him. The same process has shown that people who are depressed do in fact have negative or 'depressive' cognitions. Some experts have made the provocative suggestion, yet to be adequately tested, that faulty cognitions are *less* common among those who are depressed than in other people. According to this view, those who are *not* depressed are unduly optimistic in their appraisal of themselves and their world.

Seeing everything around us in negative terms sets up a vicious circle. Not only do negative cognitions maintain depression, but depressed mood also increases negative cognitions. When we are depressed, we tend to remember negative or unhappy memories more easily than others. Research provides good evidence of this. For example, in one study, individuals were presented with a series of words which are emotionally neutral (like 'stone' and 'mist') and asked to recall a real-life experience associated with each word. After briefly describing the particular memory recalled, the participants in the study were asked to rate each experience recalled for its pleasantness and its happiness. A larger percentage of the experiences recalled by depressed people were unhappy or unpleasant compared with those recalled by non-depressed subjects. What is more, the evidence from such studies indicates that the more severely depressed we become, the greater the proportion of memories we recall that are sad. As we recover from depression, so pleasant memories are more readily recalled and there is a corresponding decline in the recall of sad memories. It is also interesting to note that some researchers have described different patterns of cognitive distortion in men and women. A recent study of a group of American college students reported that men show greater cognitive distortion than women while at the same time having lower levels of depression. Also, the extent of this cognitive distortion was a far better predictor of depression in women than in men. These results led the researchers to suggest that the cognitive theory of depression which we outlined above describes what happens to women who become depressed, but may not apply to men. Perhaps cognitive distortion even protects men from becoming depressed. Results like these serve as a reminder of the complexity of depression and its associations.

Such evidence allows us to see how depression may be maintained by abnormal cognitions and forms the rationale for cognitive therapy in depression. However, Beck's theory goes further than this and asserts that abnormal cognitions not only maintain depression, but they may also be its actual cause. In other words, this theory sees an alteration of cognition as the primary change in depression, the change on which all others depend. This idea is much more difficult to test through research. Whether depressed mood gives rise to depressive cognitions or vice versa may seem an academic argument but it is relevant to our understanding of depression and its treatment, as we shall see. Beck suggests that unhappy or distressing experiences in childhood can give rise to packages of depressive cognitions which may re-emerge in adult life at times of stress. This offers one explanation why one of our friends may become depressed in response to a given event, while we ourselves may have a different response. An important implication of this idea is that cognitive therapy should potentially be capable of more than merely relieving the immediate symptoms of depression. Because such therapy teaches the individual to recognise and modify abnormal cognitions, it should also reduce the likelihood of further episodes of depression in the future. Future research will tell us if this is actually true.

It is not difficult to recognise the similarities between this model and the observations of Brown and Harris, already mentioned. In keeping with Brown and Harris' findings, cognitive theory predicts that the way a person construes a life event is more important than the nature of the event itself in determining whether depression will result. At least some of the vulnerability factors described by Brown and his colleagues may relate to the development of negative packages of cognitions. Thus, for example, the loss of a parent in childhood (one of Brown and Harris' vulnerability factors, referred to above) may generate negative cognitions which can become active again in adulthood when the individual is threatened with another significant loss. In our own experience as doctors, we have observed that, among those people whose emotional reactions to physical illness are particularly severe, many have had major losses or disappointments in childhood. Numerous research studies have considered this problem, with conflicting results. On present evidence, the relationship between parental separation in childhood and adult depression appears to be weak and non-specific. This does not mean it should be discounted – this association may be important in *some* depressed people but not in others.

Psychodynamic factors

So far, we have considered causes of depression (or, more correctly, *aspects* of depression) which have been tested through research, or are amenable to such testing. Even though psychodynamic principles are widely acknowledged as important in our overall understanding of depression, such ideas are very much more difficult to test by conventional scientific means. As we are mainly concerned here with research into depression, a comprehensive review of psychodynamic formulations of depression goes beyond our brief. However, we shall consider some aspects of psychodynamic thinking about depression which relate to the ideas we have already presented.

Psychodynamic thinking about depression has undoubtedly been profoundly influenced by Freud's ideas. Some of these were taken up by later writers, many of whom have emphasised that the predisposition to depression stems from experiences in early childhood, notably from the quality of the relationship between the child and its mother. An infant has no idea of 'self' and 'other' and forms a very primitive attachment to its mother, viewing her as an extension of itself. As children develop emotionally, they go through a complex phase in which they begin to recognise mother as a separate person, different from themselves. Furthermore, mother is seen as the source of both good and bad experiences (not being instantly on hand when the infant starts crying would be an example of the latter). The child also realises that his destructive impulses may harm the object he loves and upon which he is totally dependent. The mother's attitudes and behaviour are, of course, very important here — the child's successful negotiation of this stage of development depends on what Winnicott has termed 'good enough mothering'. With 'good enough mothering', the child's attachment to its mother matures through the development within itself of an image of its mother, an internal 'good object'. Once this has happened, the child no longer needs to see or touch its mother to know she exists and cares. The mother can leave her child's sight without the child fearing she has gone forever. This not only forms the 'model' for future attachments but also affects the development of the child's self-esteem.

If we fail, for whatever reason, to negotiate this process successfully, we are likely to re-enact our inadequacies in subsequent attachments we make. As Anthony Storr has expressed it: 'Diabetics who cannot manufacture their own insulin require injections of it. Depressives, who have no inner source of self-esteem, require repeated injections of reassurance, love and success to maintain emotional stability.' Melanie Klein believed that children should have worked through the difficult phase at a very early age. However, some writers dispute whether the conflicts described above are ever totally resolved. It is intriguing to speculate that all this might therefore tie in with Brown and Harris' work — in particular, with their observation that loss of mother before the age of 11 years acted as a vunerability factor in depression. Perhaps, as some have suggested, this has an enduring influence on self-esteem and on the capacity to sustain loss.

Psychodynamic theories relate mainly to processes which are unconscious, hidden far beyond our immediate awareness. Gaining access to our unconscious is often complex and difficult, requiring the use of techniques like psychoanalysis. This seems very different from cognitive theory which, as we have said, has to do with conscious processes. Even if we are not always aware of our cognitions, they are quite easily accessible to us — we can train ourselves to pay more attention to them. Cognitive theory does not even require the existence of any unconscious mechanisms. However, these differences between cognitive and psychodynamic frameworks may in the end prove more apparent than real. It is not hard to imagine, for example, that unconscious processes such as those just outlined could contribute to the depressive cognitive schemata described by Beck.

What causes depression?

Centuries ago, the name given to depression was *melancholia*; this literally means 'black bile', which was at that time thought to be the cause of depression. Since then, as our review of recent research illustrates, our knowledge and understanding of depression has become much more sophisticated. We have outlined a variety of ways of looking at depression and its associations. At first glance, it may seem that these different models of depression — biological, psychological and so on — are quite unrelated to one another. However, with the growth of our understanding through research, more and more links are emerging between these apparently disparate models.

The idea of searching for the modern equivalent of 'black bile', *the* underlying cause of depression, has lost all attraction. Instead, depression is seen as a condition with a multitude of associations — biological, psychological and social. Some of these will turn out to be causes of depression, others its effects. Each forms a piece in a complex jigsaw which when complete will afford better understanding of depression. Along with better understanding comes the possibility of better treatments, including prevention. We look forward to the time when alternative medicine will be able to contribute its share of pieces in the complex puzzle.

Addresses of Self-help and Information Services

All the organisations listed below will be able to answer questions concerning the registration of individual practitioners, or to recommend a therapist. Organisations marked with a * *only* recommend medically qualified practitioners.

**The Faculty of Homoeopathy*
The Royal London Homoeopathic Hospital
Great Ormond Street
London WC1N 3HR

**British Medical Acupuncture Society*
67–9 Chancery Lane
London WC2 1AF

British Acupuncture Association
34 Alderney Street
London SW1B 4EU

The College of Traditional Chinese Acupuncture
Tao House
Queensway
Royal Leamington Spa
Warwickshire CV31 3LZ

General Council and Register of Osteopaths
1–4 Suffolk Street
London SW1Y 4HG

British Chiropractors Association
5 First Avenue
Chelmsford
Essex CM1 1RX

Action Against Allergy
Head Office
43 The Downs
London SW20 8HG

Food Allergy Association
9 Mill Lane
Shoreham-by-Sea
West Sussex

**British Society for Nutritional Medicine*
Dr S. Davies
9 Portland Road
East Grinstead
West Sussex RH19 4EB

**British Society of Medical and Dental Hypnosis*
42 Links Road
Ashtead
Surrey KT21 2HJ

Yoga Biomedical Trust
PO Box 140
Cambridge

MIND
National Association for Mental Health
39 Queen Anne Street
London W1M 0AJ

Australia

Association of Relatives and Friends of the Mentally Ill
311 Hay Street
Subiaco
W Australia 6008

Biofeedback Meditation and Relaxation Centre
165 Adderton Road
Carlingford
NSW 2118

Acupuncture Association of Australia
1 Palmer Street
North Parramatta
NSW 2151

Homoeopathic Association of Australia
7 Hampden Road
Artarmon
NSW 2064

Australian Natural Therapies Association
729 Burwood Road
Hawthorn

Australian Osteopathic Association
71 Collins Street
Melbourne 3000

Australian Chiropractors, Osteopaths and Natural Physicians Association
6/102 Kirribilli Avenue
Kirribilli
NSW

Help Call Service
1A Hamilton Street
Mont Albert
Victoria
NSW 3127

Canada

Canadian Mental Health Association
National Office
2160 Yonge Street
Toronto
Ontario M4S 2Z3

Acupuncture Association of Canada
10 St Mary Street
Toronto
Ontario M4Y 1P9

Federation of Ontario Yoga Teachers
30 Erskine Avenue
Apartment 911
Toronto
Ontario M4P 1Y6

Canadian Association for Preventative and Orthomolecular Medicine
2177 Park Crescent
Coquitlam
British Columbia
Canada V3J 6T1

Canadian Society of Homoeopathy
Post Box 4333
Station 'E'
Ottawa
Ontario K1S 5B3

Canadian Osteopathic Association
575 Waterloo Street
London
Ontario
Canada N6B 2R2

Canadian Chiropractice Association
1900 Batview Avenue
Toronto 17
Ontario

South Africa

South African Association of Health Services
PO Box 17055
Groenkloof 0027
Pretoria
(Has details of several available therapies)

South African Homoeopathic Association
PO Box 10255
1570 Strubenvale

Chiropractice Association of South Africa
Poynton House 701
Gardiner Street
4000 Durban

USA

American Guild of Hypnotherapists
7117 Farnam Street
Omaha
Nebraska 68132

Foundation for Depression and Manic Depression
Seven E 67th Street
New York
NY 10021

Acupuncture International Association
2330 S Brentwood Boulevard
St Louis
MO 63144

Further Reading

Chapter One

Accounts of depression particularly suitable for the lay reader include:

Dominion J., *Depression: What is it? How do we cope*? (London: Fontana, 1976).
Mitchell, R., *Depression* (Harmondsworth: Penguin/MIND, 1975).
Watts, C. A. H., *Defeating Depression – A Guide for Depressed People and Their Families* (Wellingborough: Thorsons, 1980).
Winokour, G., *Depression – The Facts* (Oxford: Oxford University Press, 1981).

The British Medical Association also have two relevant booklets in their 'Family Doctor' series: Hinton, J., *Coping With Depression* and Casson, F.R.C., *Anxiety, Nervousness and Depression*.

The American Psychiatric Association's *Pyschiatric Glossary* provides useful definitions of psychiatric terms (published by the American Psychiatric Association, 1984).

Models of mental illness and psychiatric diagnosis are lucidly discussed in: Clare, A., *Psychiatry in Dissent: Controversial Issues in Thought and Practice*, 2nd ed., (London: Tavistock, 1980).

For a historical introduction to the concepts of depression, see: Lewis, A. J., 'Melancholia: a historical review', in *The State of Psychiatry: Essays and Addresses* (London: Routledge & Kegan Paul, 1967), pp. 71–110.

Any psychiatric textbook will offer an overview of depression from the psychiatric perspective. Particularly recommended is: Gelder, M., Gath, D. and Mayou, R., *Oxford Textbook of Psychiatry* (Oxford: Oxford University Press, 1983). For a more detailed account, see: Paykel E. S. (ed.), *Handbook of Affective Disorders* (Edinburgh: Churchill Livingstone, 1982).

The following deal with particular features of depression and their importance in diagnosis:

Freud, S. (1917), 'Mourning and melancholia', in Strachey, J. (ed.), *The Standard Edition of the Complete Psychological Works of Sigmund Freud*, vol. 14 (London: Hogarth Press, 1957), pp. 239–58.

Lewis, A. J., 'Melancholia; a clinical survey of depressive states', *Journal of Mental Science*, 1934, Vol. 80, pp. 277–80.
Paykel, E. S., Norton, K. R. W., 'Masked depression', *British Journal of Hospital Medicine*, 1982, vol. 28, pp. 151–7.
Freeling, P., Rao, B. M., Paykel, E. S., Sireling, L. I. and Burton, R. H., 'Contemporary themes: unrecognized depression in general practice', *British Medical Journal*, 1985, Vol. 290, pp. 1880–3.

Chapter Two

Most of the introductory accounts of depression mentioned above give accounts of the treatments used for depression. For the reader who wants more detailed information and a way into the research literature, the following selection of references may be helpful.

Placebo effects

Shapiro, A. K., 'The placebo response', in Howells, J. G. (ed.), *Modern Perspectives in World Psychiatry*, (Edinburgh: Oliver & Boyd, 1968), pp. 596–619.
Sato, T. L., Turnbull, C. D., Davidson, J. R. T. and Madakasira, S., 'Depressive illness and placebo response', in *International Journal of Psychiatry in Medicine*, 1984; vol. 14, pp. 171–9.

Drugs

British National Formulary, Number 9, British Medical Association and The Pharmaceutical Society of Great Britain, 1985.
Silverstone, T. and Turner, P., *Drug Treatment in Psychiatry*, 2nd ed. (London: Routledge & Kegan Paul, 1978).
Morgan, H. G., 'Do minor affective disorders need medication?' *British Medical Journal*, 1984, Vol. 289, p. 783.
Catalan, J. and Gath, D., 'Benzodiazepines in general practice: time for a decision', *British Medical Journal*, 1985, Vol. 290, pp. 1374–6.

Psychotherapies

Brown, D. and Pedder, J., *Introduction to Psychotherapy: An Outline of Psychodynamic Principles and Practice* (London: Tavistock, 1979).
Karasu, T. B., 'Psychotherapies: an overview,' *American Journal of Psychiatry*, 1977, Vol. 134, pp. 851–63.
Corney, R. H., 'The effectiveness of attached social workers in the management of depressed female patients in general practice', *Psychological Medicine*, Monograph Supplement 6 (Cambridge: Cambridge University Press, 1984).
DiMascio, A., Weissman, M. M., Prusoff, B. A., Neu, C., Zwilling, M.

and Klerman, G. L., 'Differential symptom reduction by drugs and psychotherapy in acute depression', *Archives of General Psychiatry*, 1979, vol. 36, pp. 1450–6.

Editorial, 'Psychotherapy: effective treatment or expensive placebo?' *The Lancet*, 1984, no. i, pp. 83–4.

Williams, J. M. G., review article, 'Cognitive-behaviour therapy for depression: problems and perspectives', *British Journal of Psychiatry*, 1984, Vol. 145, pp. 254–62.

Chapter Three

Fulder, S., *The Handbook of Complementary Medicine* (London: Coronet Books, 1984).

Chapter Four

Anon., *Essentials of Chinese Acupuncture* (Peking: Foreign Language Press, 1980).

Lu, Gwei-Djen and Needham, J., *Celestial Lancets* (Cambridge: Cambridge University Press, 1980).

Chapter Five

Blackie, M. G., *The Challenge of Homoeopathy: The Patient Not the Cure* (London: Unwin Paperbacks, 1984).

Boyd, H. W., *Introduction to Homoeopathic Medicine* (Beaconsfield: Beaconsfield Publishers, 1981).

Chapter Six

Airola, P., *Hypoglycaemia: A Better Approach* (Arizona: Health Plus Publishers, 1977).

Bland, J., *Hair Tissue Mineral Analysis* (Wellingborough: Thorsons, 1983).

Lesser, M., *Nutrition and Vitamin Therapy* (New York: Grove Press, 1980).

Lessof, M. H. (ed.), *Clinical Reactions to Food* (Chichester: John Wiley, 1983).

Randolph, T. G. and Moss, R. W., *Allergies* (London: Turnstone Press, 1981).

Rippere, V., *The Allergy Problem* (Wellingborough: Thorsons, 1983).

Chapter Seven

Ambrose, G. and Newbold, G., *A Handbook of Medical Hypnosis* (Eastbourne: Baillière Tindall, 1980).
Shaw, L. H., *Hypnosis in Practice* (Eastbourne: Baillière Tindall, 1977).
Waxman, D., *Hypnosis* (London: Allen & Unwin, 1981).

Chapter Eight

Barlow, W., *The Alexander Principle* (London: Gollancz, 1973).

Chapter Nine

For an overview of this field, the reader might find it helpful to look at: Richter, D. (ed.), *Research in Mental Illness* (London: Heinemann, 1984). A good account of some aspects of psychiatric research may be found in: Tsuang, M. T. and Vandermey, R., *Genes and the Mind* (New York: Oxford University Press, 1980).

A more detailed review of many aspects of research in depression may be found in: Gilbert, P., *Depression: From Psychology to Brain State* (London: Lawrence Erlbaum Associates, 1984). This is particularly recommended for Paul Gilbert's excellent attempt to integrate the different models of depression.

The following references offer more detailed accounts of some of the research discussed in this section:

Abramson, L. T., Seligman, M. E. P. and Teasdale, J. D., 'Learned helplessness in humans: critique and reformulation', *Journal of Abnormal Psychology*, 1978, vol. 87, pp. 49–74.
Beck, A. T., *Depression: Clinical, Experimental and Theoretical Aspects*, (New York: Harper & Row, 1967).
Beck, A. T., *Cognitive Therapy and the Emotional Disorders* (New York: International Universities Press, 1976).
Brown, G. W. and Harris, T., *The Social Origins of Depression: A Study of Psychiatric Disorder in Women* (London: Tavistock, 1978).
Calloway, S. P., 'Endocrine changes in depression', *Hospital Update*, 1982, pp. 1343–50.
Charney, D. S., Menkes, D. B., and Henniger, G. R., 'Receptor sensitivity and the mechanism of action of antidepressant treatment', *Archives of General Psychiatry*, 1981, vol. 38, pp. 1160–80.
Clare, A. W., 'Hormones, behaviour and the menstrual cycle', *Journal of Psychosomatic Research*, 1985, vol. 29, pp. 225–33.
Depue, R. A., Evans, R., 'The psychobiology of depressive disorders:

from pathophysiology to predisposition', *Progress in Experimental Personality Research*, 1981, vol. 10, pp. 1–114.

Dolan, R. J., Calloway, S. P., Fonagy, P., De Souza, F. V. A. and Wakeling, A., 'Life events, depression and hypothalamic-pituitary-adrenal axis function', *British Journal of Psychiatry*, 1985, Vol. 147, pp. 429–33.

Jesberger, J. A. and Richardson, J. S., 'Animal models of depression: parallels and correlates to severe depression in humans', *Biological Psychiatry*, 1985, vol. 20, pp. 764–84.

Kraemer, G. W., 'The primate social environment, brain neurochemical changes and psychopathology', *Trends in Neurological Sciences*, 1985, vol. 11, pp. 339–40.

Metz, A., Stump, K., Cowen, P. J., Elliott, J. M., Gelder, M. G. and Grahame-Smith, D. G., 'Changes in platelet alpha-2 adrenoceptor binding post partum: possible relation to maternity blues', *Lancet*, 1983, no. i, pp. 495–8.

Pedder, J. R., 'Failure to mourn, and melancholia', *British Journal of Psychiatry*, 1982, Vol. 141, 329–37.

Reveley, A. and Murray, R. M., 'The genetic contribution to the functional psychoses', *British Journal of Hospital Medicine*, 1980, vol. 24, pp. 166–71.

Sowa, C. J. and Lustman, P. J., 'Gender differences in rating stressful events, depression, and depressive cognition', *Journal of Clinical Psychology*, 1984, vol. 40, pp. 1334–7.

Teasdale, J. D., 'Changes in cognition during depression — psychopathological implications: discussion paper, *Journal of the Royal Society of Medicine*, 1983, vol. 76, pp. 1038–44.

Ullah, P., Banks, M. and Warr, P., 'Social support, social pressures and psychological distress during unemployment', *Psychological Medicine*, 1985, vol. 15, pp. 283–95.

Van Praag, H. M., 'Depression', *Lancet*, 1982, no. ii, pp. 1259–64.

Weissman, M. M., Klerman, G. L., 'Sex differences in the epidemiology of depression', *Archives of General Psychiatry*, 1977, vol. 34, pp. 98–111.

Index